Neuros
for
Basic Surgical Trainees

W. Adriaan Liebenberg
MB ChB (Stellenbosch), FC Neurosurg (SA)
and
Reuben D. Johnson
BSc, MB ChB (Glasg.), MRCS Glasg., MRCS Eng.

Foreword by Carl Hardwidge
BM, FRCS

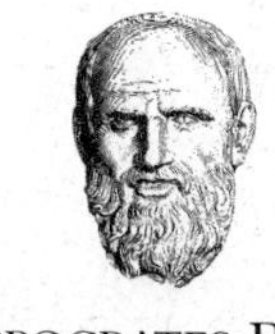

HIPPOCRATES BOOKS

8 Queen's Square, Kirkby Lonsdale, Cumbria, LA6 2AZ, UK

ISBN 0-9547314-0-9

Typeset by The Drawing Room Design Ltd., Over Kellet, Carnforth, Lancashire, UK
Printed and bound by Polestar Wheatons, Exeter, Devon, UK

CONTENTS

FOREWORD

At the start, a Senior House Officer's job in neurosurgery is daunting; nevertheless I remember my first day with some degree of affection – after all, it started me on the first steps of my soon to be chosen career. I also remember the considerable anxiety I felt. It was lucky that I had an infinitely patient Senior Registrar who held my hand until I had gained sufficient knowledge and experience to become a useful member of the team. This book will not stop any sensible SHO or newly appointed Registrar from being anxious in his or her new job, but it will give them access to an infinitely patient Senior Registrar who has the advantage of being constantly accessible and fits into their white coat pocket. Liebenberg and Johnson have managed to produce a text that is a working man's guide to day-to-day practical neurosurgery. They have combined discursive passages with a quick guide, which allows instant access to the information needed to run a neurosurgical ward on a day-to-day basis. I congratulate them on their efforts. I believe this book will be standard equipment for the new SHO and Registrar in neurosurgery.

Carl Hardwidge BM, FRCS
Consultant Neurosurgeon
Lead Clinician, Hurstwood Park Neurological Centre
STC Chairman (South Thames)
Examiner for Intercollegiate Fellowship in Neurosurgery

PREFACE

The management of neurosurgical patients can appear complex and daunting to the basic surgical trainee. The extra responsibility required to undertake the ward management of these patients is reflected by the exclusion of junior house officers from neurosurgical posts. Unfortunately, due to the recent reduction in junior doctors' hours there has been a proportionate and dramatic reduction in training opportunities. There is a specific need, therefore, for a pocket text that will guide the basic surgical trainee through the essentials of managing neurosurgical patients. This volume has been written specifically for the trainee starting their first neurosurgical post. It is hoped that this text will serve as a guide to senior house officers (SHOs) during the first few weeks of their job. The rudiments of a neurosurgical history and examination are covered, and an overview of neurosurgical pathology is given. Advice and tips are given on the management of emergency admissions and elective neurosurgical patients. The basics of interpreting neurosurgical CT scans are described succinctly. The fundamentals of the more common and standard neurosurgical procedures are described – from burr-holes to trauma craniotomy, from external ventricular drains to ventriculoperitoneal shunts. An overview of the use of neuro-ICU is given and an approach to neuro-ICU patients outlined. To help SHOs make the most of their time in neurosurgery, and to facilitate their discussions with senior colleagues, a chapter is included which overviews some of the controversies and evidence base in neurosurgery.

W. Adriaan Liebenberg and Reuben D. Johnson, 2004

ACKNOWLEDGEMENTS

We are indebted to Mr Hardwidge for his help and advice and for writing the foreword to this book. We are also most grateful to Mr Norris for his expertise and guidance with the early drafts. We should also like to thank Professor Hartzenberg of Stellenbosch University, whose enthusiasm in teaching has been such a great inspiration to so many neurosurgeons. We are most grateful to everyone in the Hurstwood Park team with whom it has been a great pleasure to work. In particular, we are most grateful to the following people for their help in the work with this book: Dr Olney, Dr Good and Lynn for help with the angiograms; and Pete Foster for producing some of the photographs. We are exceptionally grateful to Carl Zeiss Ltd who have made the production of this book possible by providing us with an educational grant.

W. Adriaan Liebenberg and Reuben D. Johnson, 2004

1

Duties and Responsibilities of the Neurosurgical SHO

CONTENTS

OVERVIEW AND GENERAL DUTIES

It seems that there are several reasons that people elect to undertake a Senior House Office (SHO) post in neurosurgery. There are those who, quite rightly, are fascinated by the human nervous system and wish to become neurosurgeons. Others wish to become ophthalmologists or orthopaedic surgeons and feel that some exposure to neurosurgery is valuable experience for their chosen specialties. Then there are those who obtained neurosurgical posts as part of a wider basic surgical rotation. Whatever the reasons for doing the job, however, it is to be hoped that people will endeavour to get as much out of the job as possible. If things are organized properly by the SHOs, there are plenty of opportunities to go to theatre and outpatients, and it is in these two places that neurosurgery really comes to life. The neurosurgical Intensive Care Unit (ICU) is often blocked with the very poorly patients with a poor outcome. However, these patients are not a real reflection of the workload of the department – you need to get to theatre and see the follow-ups in clinic to see what neurosurgery can really achieve.

The duties of the neurosurgical SHO primarily consist of taking care of the ward and running the pre-op clinics. Occasionally, when things are busy, it may be necessary to carry the Registrar's receiving bleep. This is an excellent opportunity to learn and can make for an interesting day – provided it isn't an everyday occurrence! A small section on how to take neurosurgical referrals is included at the end of this chapter.

ORGANIZATION OF THE WORKING DAY

In most units, the day begins with a morning meeting similar to the trauma meeting in an orthopaedic unit. The format differs between units but usually will consist of the SHO and Registrar on-call overnight presenting new admissions and referrals. Both SHO and Registrar may be asked detailed questions by the Consultants on the history, examination and scans of the previous day's admissions. Questions usually follow on the management options. This is an excellent forum in which to learn about neurosurgery and the opportunity should be taken to ask questions of the Consultants, especially on more controversial issues. If it is found that things are getting a bit routine at the meeting, then it is worth presenting patients before putting the scan up to see whether people can diagnose and locate lesions on the basis of history and examination.

After the meeting, the morning round will probably begin on the ICU and this will led by the neurosurgical Registrars and anaesthetic team. This is a relatively easy part of the day for the SHO as the ICU staff will gather all relevant results for the round. However, it is essential that the SHO understands what is happening and the management plans, as they will probably be bleeped during the day to deal with any problems. The SHOs usually write in the notes on the ICU round. Care should be taken to document the diagnosis, any surgery so far, and number of days post-op, the neurological status (Glasgow Coma Scale [GCS] score, pupillary response, focal deficits), cardiorespiratory status (use of inotropes, type of respiratory support and percentage oxygen), evidence of any infection, and a management plan for the day. The management plan should be a clearly numbered list, e.g.: (1) computerized tomography (CT) scan tomorrow; (2) if no changes on CT, wean sedation and reassess neurology; (3) keep intracranial pressure (ICP) $<20\,cmH_2O$ until sedation weaned.

The round will progress to the ward and, ideally, the SHOs should present each patient, i.e., name, age, diagnosis, procedure, and progress. Nursing staff should be given the opportunity to raise any issues. Checklists for each type of patient are given in the later chapter on the ward management of neurosurgical patients. However, it is worth bearing a few matters in mind at this point. It is essential to check wounds frequently for signs of infection or cerebrospinal fluid (CSF) leak. Obviously, blood results should be available for the round, and particular attention should be paid to reporting daily sodium levels for patients with subarachnoid haemorrhage (SAH) and for patients after pituitary surgery. For patients with tumours, steroids should be reviewed each day to ensure that there is a plan in place for their discontinuation. Patients are rarely discharged on steroids, though a small maintenance dose may be given to tumour patients until they are seen by the oncologist, or to pituitary patients until they are seen by the endocrinologist. We make no apologies for repeating the point: never let a patient leave the unit without a plan to stop their steroids, and for someone to check this at a suitable date. It is advisable to be up-to-date on histology results and know when they are due, and to ensure that there are dates for oncology or endocrinology review.

Following the round, the ward jobs tend to consist of ordering scans and referring patients back to their local hospitals. Some units allow letters to be dictated, whereas in others letters will have to be typed by the SHOs. It is best if the SHO team can find an efficient way of organizing referrals back. Valuable information often goes missing and so, if possible, document the name of the Consultant who referred the patient to the neurosurgical patient early on. Letters to the local hospital should include a summary of the presentation, details of the procedure, progress so far, a brief note about expected prognosis, details of medication (including plans to stop steroids), and arrangements for follow-up. Remember that many tumour biopsies are taken in the neurosurgical unit to provide a diagnosis so that definitive treatment can be planned and administered elsewhere.

Once all the ward jobs have been completed (hopefully by mid-morning!) the rest of the day will consist of covering the ward and ICU, seeing any new admissions, theatre, or pre-op assessment. If there is no afternoon round by the Registrar on-call, it might be useful for the SHOs to get together before the end of office hours (e.g., 4 p.m.-ish) to check that all results are back and acted upon. Ensure that any scans ordered have been done and seen, and decisions made by the Registrar or Consultant. It is the responsibility of the person who signs the request form to make sure that the scans are reviewed – so if you sign it, make sure you see the scan and show it to someone who can make a decision.

Pre-op clinics are pretty much the same as in other specialties. Assessments are made for fitness for surgery and relevant investigations organized. It is essential to ensure that anticoagulants and aspirin are discontinued in good time before most neurosurgical procedures. Most Consultants prefer patients to be off all forms of NSAID at least a week prior to elective surgery, particularly for intradural procedures whether cranial or spinal.

In neurosurgery, SHOs do not carry their own receiving bleep, are not asked to go to A&E, and are usually only required to attend a few outpatient clinics. This should make the job less hectic than general surgical or orthopaedic jobs. Some regard their neurosurgical SHO job as being like another house-officer post. However, the neurosurgical SHO post requires a higher level of responsibility and knowledge than a house job. If the SHOs work as a team, then everyone should be able to spend at least one or two days per week in theatre. There is ample opportunity to get hands on drills!

TAKING NEUROSURGICAL REFERRALS

Taking neurosurgical referrals is unlike taking referrals in most other surgical specialties you will have worked in. You will not always be able to walk down to the Accident and Emergency (A&E) department to see what is actually going on, because frequently the patient will be miles away in another hospital. Despite this, you may find that, once you have been phoned, the person making the referral will assume you have taken over the care of the patient! There is also a widespread assumption among referring specialties that all you need is the scans. *Never* accept a referral of the 'Have you seen Mr Thompson's scans? Are you going take him?' Assume that, in such cases, Mr Thompson has fixed dilated pupils, a massive diffuse head injury, a clam-shell thoracotomy (but no IV access), bilateral open femoral shaft fractures, and has not had any C-spine films.

Whilst this may seem obvious, the importance of obtaining as much of the relevant information as possible at the time of the first call cannot be overemphasized. If the person referring can't answer all your questions, make sure they understand that advice can only be given once all the information is available. Remember to be polite: neurosurgical cases can be quite frightening, especially to the uninitiated, and we can all forget things in a crisis. By all means look at the scans and present them to your Registrar, but make it clear that the referring team is gathering all the facts. The following is the minimum amount of information that should be obtained from the referring team. *Don't accept anything less!*

DETAILS OF THE REFERRING TEAM

Name of referring doctor
Contact number of referring doctor
Name of Consultant in charge in referring hospital
Name of referring hospital

It cannot be overemphasized how important these details are. It is all too easy to put the phone down after obtaining a great history only to find you don't know which hospital the patient is in! Beware the 5 p.m. referral. The referring doctor might be going off-duty. Make sure to ask and that you know the contact details of their replacement.

PATIENT DETAILS

Name
Age
Date of birth
Location (A&E/ward)

Remember that A&E departments can be quite big. If a patient is comatose in A&E don't just assume they are in resuscitation!

HISTORY

Sequence of events
Past medical history
Drug history
Social history

Obtain a concise sequence of events and begin to formulate a picture in your mind as to what sort of pathology you might be dealing with (see Chapter 4, on history and examination). Tailor questions according to pathology; e.g., if the history sounds spinal make sure to enquire about sphincter control. When the history is equivocal always enquire regarding a history of trauma (e.g., subarachnoids can be traumatic as well as spontaneous). If there is trauma, are there any other injuries? In the case of the comatose patient ask about medically reversible causes (e.g., fits, blood sugar). Past medical history and drug history are very important. If someone has a tumour on their scan it is nice to know whether they have a known lung primary. Similarly, if someone has had an acute subdural haemorrhage (ASDH), it is useful to know that they have atrial fibrillation (AF) and are on 5 mg of warfarin. Brief social history should be obtained along the lines of an orthopaedic-type social history, including details about mobility, e.g., 'Mrs Jones lives in a warden-controlled residential home, uses two sticks to walk, but is otherwise independent and takes the bus to go shopping'.

EXAMINATION

Current GCS	Peripheral deficits
Any fluctuations in GCS	Reflexes
Pupils: size and reaction	Sphincters
Cranial nerve abnormalities	Observations (obs)

Certain parts of the GCS may be more relevant than others; e.g., best motor response (see Chapter 4, on history and examination). Always make sure, therefore, that the person referring can break down the GCS into all its components and ask them what they mean – do not accept '$E_1V_3M_4$'! You need to ask them to tell you in words what the eyes, speech, and motor response actually are. Ask about fluctuations in the GCS: it might be 13 but it also may keep dropping down to 5. Pupil size and reaction need to be documented even if the GCS is 15, as pupil dilatation due to tentorial herniation can occur in the awake patient. Deficits in cranial nerve territory and peripheral nervous system help localize pathology. Sphincter assessment again is necessary if a compressive spinal lesion is suspected. Always take a note of the obs to include pulse, blood pressure, haemoglobin oxygen saturation (sats) and temperature. Always be thinking about whether the examination is consistent with the history. For example, a history of fits and confusion does not necessarily fit with a GCS of 15.

MANAGEMENT IN THE REFERRING HOSPITAL

Location of patient ABCs and advanced trauma life support (ATLS) Investigations Treatments Most senior doctor/Consultant's opinion

Make sure you know or enquire about the location of the patient. Remember that at this stage you are only taking a referral and are not managing the patient. However, if it sounds as though the patient needs to be in a high-dependency area, then suggest that this is discussed in the referring hospital. Are you happy with the airway? If a patient has a GCS less than 8 suggest that the referring team needs to speak to the anaesthetist in their hospital as intubation might be appropriate. Don't insist dogmatically on intubation at this stage unless it is obvious that the patient will need transferring. Remember, the patient may have had a pre-terminal event and intubation may be entirely inappropriate. If there is a history of trauma, has the full ATLS protocol been carried out? Enquire about what investigations have been undertaken and what is being sent to you. For example, have the scans been linked? In trauma, have C-spine films been undertaken? If there is a suspected tumour, what investigations have been undertaken to hunt for a possible primary? Make sure you find out what treatments have been initiated in the referring hospital (e.g., steroids, mannitol).

PLAN

You should always discuss the plan before you put the phone down. This might be that you will discuss the case and scans with your Registrar or Consultant and get back to them. However, it might be that the referring team initiates some further investigations or gets an anaesthetist involved.

WRITE IT DOWN

You may have got it all down into the book first time or jotted notes on the first available piece of paper. Make sure you write it all down in the book before you hand it over to someone else.

2

Overview of Neurosurgical Patients

CONTENTS

INTRODUCTION

Neurosurgery, like all other specialties, is divided into subgroups. It will be helpful when starting an SHO post to have some understanding of these subdivisions and to be aware where the interests of the Consultants in your unit lie. The subdivisions are listed below with a brief description of each.

VASCULAR NEUROSURGERY

Vascular neurosurgeons treat patients who have vascular abnormalities, such as arteriovenous malformations (AVMs), aneurysms, dural arteriovenous fistulas, or cavernomas; they may also carry out surgery involving the carotid or, rarely, bypass surgery.

PITUITARY NEUROSURGERY

Pituitary neurosurgeons treat hormone-secreting pituitary adenomas with surgery in cases where medical therapy has failed, or space-occupying non-hormone-producing adenomas with the aim of preventing blindness and of reducing compression of brain tissue.

SKULL-BASE NEUROSURGERY

Skull-base neurosurgeons treat skull-base tumours on the clivus, dorsum sellae, in the cerebellopontine angle, around the third ventricle, foramen magnum, and parasellar area

SPINAL NEUROSURGERY

Spinal neurosurgeons decompress the spinal cord and nerve roots by means of laminectomies, discectomies, foraminotomies and anterior approaches, and they fuse the vertebral column with bony fusion and instrumentation. Some spinal neurosurgeons will be involved in the treatment of developmental abnormalities and deformities of the spine.

PAEDIATRIC NEUROSURGERY

Paediatric neurosurgeons treat pathologies similar to those in adult patients plus the developmental abnormalities seen in children (see Chapter 9, on paediatric neurosurgery).

FUNCTIONAL NEUROSURGERY

Functional neurosurgeons undertake the surgical treatment of epilepsy and movement disorders.

PAIN NEUROSURGERY

Some neurosurgeons treat neurovascular compression syndromes such as trigeminal neuralgia and hypoglossal neuralgia. They use a variety of methods, including microvascular decompression and ablative procedures. Intractable dysaesthetic pain following failed back surgery or trauma can be treated with spinal stimulators, posterior rhizotomies or stimulation/ablation of the peri-aquaductal grey area or areas of the thalamus.

TRAUMA NEUROSURGERY

Trauma neurosurgery is usually included in the repertoire of the general neurosurgeon. This includes cranial soft tissue damage, skull fracture, traumatic haemorrhage and spinal trauma

RADIOSURGERY

Oncologists and some neurosurgeons treat patients with external radiation. The Linac accelerator, which works with conventional radiation beams, and the Gamma knife (Cobalt 60 source), are two focused external radiation sources that can focus on a very small area of brain and have a minimal effect on surrounding structures.

ONCOLOGICAL NEUROSURGERY

Oncological neurosurgeons obviously treat neurological tumours and this forms a very large part of neurosurgical practice. Surgical management involves resection of tumours and biopsy for diagnostic purposes. They will collaborate closely with the oncological physicians in the management of these patients.

GENERAL NEUROSURGERY

The ambit of the general neurosurgeon is usually taken to include spinal, trauma, oncology, CSF diversion, posterior fossa surgery and peripheral nerve surgery.

3
Neurosurgical Pathology

CONTENTS

- Disorders of CSF flow
  - Obstructive (noncommunicating) hydrocephalus
  - Communicating hydrocephalus
  - Normal pressure hydrocephalus
  - Benign intracranial hypertension
  - Causes of shunt failure
- Congenital disorders presenting in adulthood
  - Aqueduct stenosis
  - Chiari malformations
    - Chiari I
    - Chiari II
- Intracranial infection

Spinal disorders
- Tumours
- Degenerative disease
- Infection
- Spinal cord syndromes
  - Syndromes of the upper spinal cord
    - Anterior spinal cord syndrome
    - Central cord syndrome
    - Bell's cruciate paralysis
  - Syndromes of the lower spinal cord
    - Conus medullaris syndrome
    - Cauda equina syndrome

Peripheral nerve disorders

CRANIAL DISORDERS

MANIFESTATIONS OF CEREBRAL DISEASE

As neurosurgeons, we deal mostly with either compressive or destructive lesions. The history usually gives an accurate idea of the type of pathology involved, and this usually is indicated by the length of the history and the progression. Patients who have sudden acute episodes with associated headache and immediate deficit or loss of consciousness, have usually had a vascular type of incident, whereas people who present with progressive mental dysfunction, speech difficulties and progressive limb deficits, usually have a tumour of some description. Sometimes, patients present with seizures alone, and this is quite typical usually of low grade tumours, or arteriovenous malformation, although this is not exclusively true. When presented with a patient who has a history of dysfunction and has clinical signs on examination, it is important to localize the lesion to the part of the CNS from which it originates. Specific lobes of the brain have specific functions.

Frontal lobes

The frontal lobes are concerned with personality, the cortical control of micturition and conjugate eye movement. The main function of the frontal lobes, however, is motor function, and the whole motor strip is found in the posterior aspect of the frontal lobe, in front of the central sulcus. Penfield's homunculus demonstrates which part of the cortex is responsible for which part of the body. A lesion on the convexity on the lateral side will cause dysfunction of the facial muscles, whereas lesions parasagittally in midline will cause dysfunction of the legs. Speech is also controlled by the lower part of the motor strip, the so-called Broca's speech area, and lesions here result in an expressive dysphasia. Seizures are common with frontal lobe lesions.

Parietal lobes

The parietal lobes are quite small; located behind the central sulcus, they are mostly concerned with recording sensory information and spatial orientation. Speech is relayed *via* the supramarginal and angular gyri. The other important part of the parietal lobes is the visual association area, governing awareness of the images recorded in the occipital lobes. Lesions in the parietal lobes therefore lead to cortical sensory loss, dysphasia in a dominant hemisphere lesion (speech is usually located in a dominant hemisphere), and dyspraxia (inability to move limbs appropriately because of a loss of spatial orientation) in a nondominant hemisphere. A parietal lesion would also lead to a homonymous hemianopia or an attention hemianopia (see Chapter 4, on examination).

Occipital lobes

The occipital lobes are truly small and are mainly concerned with visual function. Lesions in the occipital lobe lead to blindness in the contralateral eye with sparing of the pupillary reflex, which, as we shall see, loops only as far back as the brainstem.

Temporal lobes

Once again, seizures are a large part of the manifestation of temporal lobe pathology, and, as we shall see, a contralateral upper quadrant hemianopia is seen when the fibres of Meyer's loop are affected. The centre for receptive speech discrimination – Wernicke's area – is located in the superior temporal gyrus, and lesions in this area lead to receptive dysphasia. Bilateral lesions in the temporal lobe can also cause memory deficit.

Summary

- *Frontal lobes*

Motor function	Speech
Micturition	Conjugate eye movements
Personality	Higher mental function

- *Parietal lobes*
  - Sensory awareness
  - Spatial awareness (nondominant hemisphere)
  - Speech (dominant hemisphere)
  - Visual tracts
- *Occiptal lobes*
  - Vision
- *Temporal lobes*
  - Vision
  - Receptive speech

TYPES OF CENTRAL NERVOUS SYSTEM (CNS) PATHOLOGY

Having taken a full history and carried out a full examination, and having put the signs together and come to the conclusion that somebody has a cranial problem rather than a spinal problem, and then having localized the problem to a suspected lobe, we are now ready to do investigations on our patient. Once we have the results back from our investigation, we then have to put forward a differential diagnosis. This is impossible without understanding the pathology of the CNS. The main types of CNS pathology that concern neurosurgeons are: malignancy; infection; inflammation; vascular abnormalities; and abnormal CSF flow patterns.

Intracranial malignancy

There are many ways of classifying CNS tumours. Pathologically, these tumours can be classified according to cell type: e.g., glial tumours or tumours of neuroepithelial origin. However, it can be extremely useful to consider tumours according to their anatomical site of origin in the CNS. In the forebrain and cerebellum, there are tumours that are inside the parenchyma of the brain and tumours that are outside the parenchyma of the brain but still inside the cranium. The first group are known as intra-axial tumours and the second group of tumours are called extra-axial tumours. What follows here is a discussion of the types of tumour that most commonly occur in different parts of the intracranial compartment. This is not a dry and formal description of pathology *per se*. Rather, it is a more general discussion which aims to include some insights into the particular problems different tumours present to the patient and clinician. Spinal tumours are considered later.

Intra-axial tumours

The most common intra-axial tumours are metastatic tumours that have spread mostly from the lung in males and breast in females (but also from the skin, kidney, prostate). The second most common intra-axial tumours are glial cell tumours and are known as gliomas.

Metastatic tumours

Metastatic tumours are sometimes treated by surgical excision. However, they are frequently multiple, and treating the cerebral metastases does not remove the primary tumour. The exception is in patients with fully treated primary tumours and single superficial metastases; these patients are quite often offered surgery, plus adjuvant therapy. The main aim in patients with metastatic tumours is tissue diagnosis, and chest X-ray, breast examination in females, and CT scanning of the abdomen is indicated to try and find a more accessible lesion from which to obtain a tissue diagnosis. If the hunt for the primary is unsuccessful, we would then offer a stereotactic biopsy of one of the lesions which we thought would be the most accessible and least likely to lead to complications.

Glial tumours (gliomas)

Glial tumours, or gliomas, are divided into four grades by the WHO classification, the first of these being reserved for the juvenile pilocytic astrocytoma, which is a slow-growing tumour we see in children, and subependymal giant cell astrocytomas, which are intraventricular slow-growing tumours that we infrequently see in adults. Tumours are graded according to their histological characteristics, and four features are searched for: mitosis, nuclear polymorphism, neovascularity, and necrosis. Tumours which have only mitotic features or nuclear polymorphism are usually graded as Grade II, whereas where there is evidence of new blood vessel formation the tumours are usually classed as high-grade, or Grade III gliomas. Tumours where the tissue growth is so rapid that the tissue outstrips its blood supply, and therefore undergoes areas of necrosis, are by definition Grade IV tumours, also called glioblastoma multiforme (GBM). Because glial tumours are made up of brain tissue, they frequently appear as irregular bits of brain on CT scans before the administration of contrast, and in cases of low-grade tumours there is no enhancement with contrast. The one exception to this rule is the juvenile pilocytic astrocytoma, which enhances vividly, although it remains a Grade I tumour. The usual reason for enhancement of a tumour is because of the new blood vessels forming inside the tumour, and enhancement with contrast denotes a high-grade tumour. If there is added necrosis, it then becomes a fairly obvious diagnosis of glioblastoma multiforme. We therefore find that most irregular-looking enhancing tumours are either metastases (since these also have neovascularity) or high-grade gliomas. Both of these tumours carry a grim prognosis and more than 70% of patients with glioblastoma multiforme are dead within 9 months. These malignancies unfortunately are untreatable and palliation is the only option. The decision to offer a debulking procedure usually hinges on the patient's age, general condition and Karnofsky score (a score derived from patient's ability to function in everyday life – see Chapter 13, Table 7). Patients who present at an advanced stage with malignant tumours carry the worst prognosis. This is due to the fact that they are medically less fit, and also because these tumours are usually much more aggressive biologically than tumours that present in younger patients. The basis of treatment of these malignant tumours is a debulking procedure without damage to normal brain, followed by radiotherapy. Only a single treatment of radiotherapy can be given to any one patient, and therefore regrowth after radiotherapy leaves only the option of further debulking and chemotherapy. Most patients, as noted before, do not survive very long, but there are a few notable exceptions, and therefore if patients have good Karnofsky scores and wish to have their tumours treated, they should be offered treatment.

Oligodendrogliomas

Another type of primary brain tumour is the oligodendroglioma, which is made up of oligodendrocytes. This is a slow-growing tumour, which enhances irregularly with contrast, just like the malignant tumours, but is usually found in the frontal lobes and may have lots of calcification in it. Because calcium is hyperdense like bone, tumours of this type are usually hyperdense on CT scan before contrast, and are relatively easily diagnosed. They are more benign than the malignant gliomas, and patients have been known to survive a long time with these tumours. Debulking and chemotherapy is usually indicated in the anaplastic variant with these tumours being very chemo-sensitive.

Non-Hodgkin's B-cell lymphoma

Another tumour which is hyperdense before contrast, but less intensely so, and usually located in a periventricular location, is non-Hodgkin's B-cell lymphoma. Because the brain does not have a lymphatic system, all of these are theoretically metastatic tumours, although there is a distinct difference between patients with a known systemic lymphoma and patients in whom the tumour appears to function as a primary brain tumour. These tumours are particularly common in patients with HIV-AIDS. They enhance with contrast quite uniformly. They carry quite a grim prognosis and usually need multi-modal therapy.

Intraventricular tumours

Intraventricular tumours are fairly rare, and the differential diagnosis would be tumours arising from the arachnoid cap cells (meningiomas), from the choroid plexus (papillomas or carcinomas), from the subependymal lining (subependymal giant cell astrocytomas), and from the ependyma (ependymomas). Another benign intraventricular lesion is a colloid cyst, a hyperdense cystic lesion in the third ventricle, which obstructs the foramina of Munro and can lead to sudden death. Midline tumours in the pituitary fossa and pineal region can also invade and extend into the ventricular system because of its close proximity. These are, however, extra-axial tumours.

Posterior fossa tumours

In adults, an intra-axial posterior fossa tumour is either a metastatic tumour, a haemangioblastoma, or more infrequently, a glioma. Haemangioblastomas are benign tumours, which consist of a largely cystic component and a small mural module. They can usually be excised quite successfully with surgery. In a small number of cases, a posterior fossa haemangioblastoma can be part of von Hippel Lindau syndrome. This syndrome is typified by the presence of two or more of the following:

- A positive family history of von Hippel Lindau (autosomal dominant inheritance).
- Posterior fossa haemangioblastoma.
- A retinal haemangioma.
- Renal cysts or carcinoma.
- Pancreatic cysts or carcinoma.
- Epididymal cysts.
- A phaeochromocytoma.

A small number of patients also suffer from increased red blood cell production secondary to excess erythropoietin secretion.

Extra-axial tumours

Meningiomas

Meningiomas arise from the arachnoid cap cells in the dura and are mostly benign tumours. They arise from the covering of the brain and cause symptoms and signs by compressing the brain just as an extra-axial collection of subdural or extradural blood would. They have also been called dural warts due to their appearance. These tumours are peripherally located and are diagnosed by the fact that they always have dural attachments. They are frequently very vascular and the distinguishing sign on CT scanning is that they enhance vividly with contrast. Surgery on these lesions can, therefore, frequently be quite tricky, with great blood loss. To try to prevent this they are often embolized preoperatively to reduce their vascularity.

Pituitary region tumours

Brain tumours in the pituitary region are also extra-axial, and the differential diagnosis for tumours in the pituitary region would be pituitary adenoma, metastasis, meningioma, vascular cerebral aneurysm, epidermoid tumours, germ-cell tumours, arachnoid cysts, or craniopharyngiomas.

Pituitary adenomas. Pituitary adenomas are either functional (secreting hormones) or nonfunctional (non-hormone secreting). The more usual hormone-secreting adenomas are prolactinomas, which may be microadenomas (<1 cm), mesoadenomas (1–2 cm), or macroadenomas (>2 cm).

There are also cortisol-producing adenomas (usually microadenomas), growth-hormone-producing adenomas, or thyroid-stimulating-hormone-producing adenomas.

Prolactinomas. Prolactinomas cause the clinical picture of galactorrhoea and amenorrhoea in women, and impotence and hypogonadism in men. Cortisol-producing adenomas cause Cushing's disease and growth-hormone-producing adenomas produce acromegaly in adults and gigantism in children.

Craniopharyngiomas. Craniopharyngiomas are benign lesions, which take a long time to grow but cause problems because of compression of the hypothalamus and obstruction of CSF flow. These tumours are thought to arise from remnants of Rathke's cleft, and are classified as adamantomatous or papillary. The adamantomatous type is found in children and is more aggressive; the papillary type is found in adults and is less aggressive. These tumours have an epithelial lining and enlarge slowly by the shedding of this epithelium into the cavity. The resulting keratin and cholesterol crystals cause this tumour to be different on imaging from a macroadenoma. On CT scanning, they usually have multiple areas of calcification and enhance with contrast; on magnetic resonance imaging (MRI), they have a variable appearance but are frequently hyperintense on T1 and T2, indicating not just the fluid content but also fat content due to the cholesterol crystals. Children will usually present with growth retardation, other pituitary deficiencies and visual defects. Adults are more likely to present with visual field defects and pituitary dysfunction.

Aneurysms

Aneurysms can present like tumours with mass effect, and, if they are large, they are visible on CT scanning and enhance with contrast, just as tumours would do. Taking a biopsy from an aneurysm unfortunately leads to drastic consequences and one must take care not to fall into this trap. Angiography is, therefore, a useful investigation if there is any doubt.

Pineal region tumours

Tumours in the pineal region (just posterior to the third ventricle) are either made up of the substance of the pineal gland (pinealomas and pinealoblastomas), or are germ-cell tumours. Pinealomas are tumours with fairly good prognosis. Pinealoblastomas are very aggressive tumours. Germ-cell tumours are either germinomas or teratomas, and they can frequently be diagnosed by doing serum markers for human chorionic gonadotrophin (β-HCG), fetal alkaline phosphatase or alpha-fetoprotein. They are usually extremely radiosensitive and there is also great controversy over whether they should be resected, biopsied, or whether they should undergo radiotherapy without any form of surgery.

Cerebellopontine angle tumours

Tumours in the cerebellopontine angle are either acoustic neuromas (vestibular schwannomas), meningiomas, metastases, arachnoid cysts or epidermoid tumours.

Vestibular schwannomas are nerve sheath tumours arising on the vestibular nerve; they are slow-growing, benign tumours and frequently are associated with neurofibromatosis type 1 (NF1, von Recklinghausen's disease) and neurofibromatosis type 2 (NF2). The gene for NF1 is located on chromosome 17q11.2 and codes for the protein neurofibromin. Although more than half of NF1 cases are due to an inherited autosomal dominant mutation, there is a significant proportion of sporadic new mutations. NF2 is due to inactivation of the schwannomin gene located on chromosome 22q12.2. Clinical manifestions of NF1 include: neurofibromas (commonly on skin); skin abnormalities (café au lait spots); axillary freckling; and Lisch nodules (neurofibromas on the cornea). A small number of these patients also have optic gliomas. Skin abnormalities are less common in NF2 patients, but the presence of bilateral acoustic neuromas is pathognomonic.

Vestibular schwannomas usually present with tinnitus and hearing loss; facial nerve dysfunction is, however, infrequent, even though these tumours usually compress and splay the anterior located seventh nerve during growth. In tumours smaller than 3 cm, radiosurgery can be quite successful. Patients with larger tumours usually need surgery and most surgeons will monitor small tumours for growth before planning surgery.

One controversy surrounding acoustic neuromas relates to whether they should undergo radiosurgery or open surgery. Situations where radiosurgery might be beneficial include:

- Lesions <3 cm
- Where hearing preservation is important
- Medically unfit patients
- Patients who request it.

Surgery is preferred in patients who are medically fit with large lesions, smaller tumours that are growing, or for patients who have indicated that they would prefer surgery. Another controversy is whether one should aim for a posterior fossa approach, or a translabyrinthine approach. Hearing is usually lost whichever approach is used. However, hearing preservation is normally seen when a posterior fossa approach is undertaken, or when the tumour is very small and a middle fossa approach is undertaken. A middle fossa approach is uncommon in the UK. In the proper hands, these tumours carry a very good prognosis. The main complications are postoperative facial nerve palsies, other cranial nerve damage, and CSF leaks.

Epidermoid tumours

Epidermoid tumours are inclusion tumours and they consist of epithelium. They are enclosed at the time of neural tube folding during embryogenesis and are similar to craniopharyngiomas, in the sense that they slowly enlarge because of epithelial cell desquamation. They are benign tumours but, like the craniopharyngiomas, are impossible to remove totally; luckily, however, they have a very slow growth pattern. Craniopharyngiomas and epidermoid tumours can be treated only with surgery since radiotherapy has little effect on them.

Intracranial vascular disorders

Bleeding into the cranial space frequently has disastrous consequences. Bleeding can either be intraparenchymal, or can occur in the ventricular, subarachnoid, subdural or extradural spaces. The mechanism can either be traumatic or spontaneous. It should also be borne in mind that intracranial vascular abnormalities may present without bleeding, due to their compressing local CNS structures.

Spontaneous bleeds

Cerebral aneurysms

Spontaneous bleeds are due to abnormal vasculature, and in cases of cerebral aneurysms this is due to weakness and out-pouching of the tunica interna and media through deficient external layers of the blood vessels. This is thought to be a flow-related mechanism and is usually found at vessel bifurcations at the site of the greatest flow. Because the blood vessels are located in the subarachnoid space, aneurysms usually lead to subarachnoid bleeds. There is, however, a percentage of aneurysmal bleeds that either also have a parenchymal component or are completely intraparenchymal with no subarachnoid component. Usually there has been a previous leak which has caused some fibrosis between the fundus of the aneurysm and the parenchyma, so that when this ruptures, instead of leaking into the subarachnoid space, it leaks straight into the parenchyma of the brain, presenting like a cerebrovascular accident (CVA) with a deep blood clot in the brain tissue. Aneurysms are classified according to their size, i.e., small (<10 mm), large (>10 mm), giant (>25 mm), or their location, i.e., which blood vessel they arose from (internal carotid, bifurcation, anterior communicating artery, middle cerebral artery, basilar artery, posterior cerebral artery, posterior inferior cerebellar artery, etc).

Making the diagnosis of SAH is critical, and there are two components to it. The first is identifying the blood on a CT scan, and the second is demonstrating the breakdown products of blood by spectroscopy. CT scans are 98% sensitive in the first 12 h after the ictus for detection of SAH, but decline in sensitivity after that to about 70% by day 3. It is, therefore, quite possible to miss the diagnosis if CT scans are used as the only diagnostic modality. If blood enters the CSF, the red cells lyse and oxyhaemoglobin is liberated. This is then converted to billirubin, a process which takes 12 h; this can only happen *in vivo* since the enzyme is found only in the brain itself. CSF in a test tube will therefore produce oxyhaemoglobin secondary to lysis of red blood cells, but not bilirubin because of the absence of the enzyme. The presence of bilirubin can have only one explanation: that there has been blood present in the subarachnoid space for at least 12 h, thus confirming the diagnosis of SAH. This underlies the extreme importance of waiting 12 h before doing the lumbar puncture (LP). If it is done before 12 h it will be negative for bilirubin and may allow blood to be introduced into the subarachnoid space, therefore making any further testing a futile exercise. Doing the LP more than 12 h after the ictus will make the diagnosis successfully in 100% of cases for 2 weeks. The steps involved in making a diagnosis of SAH are summarized in Figure 1.

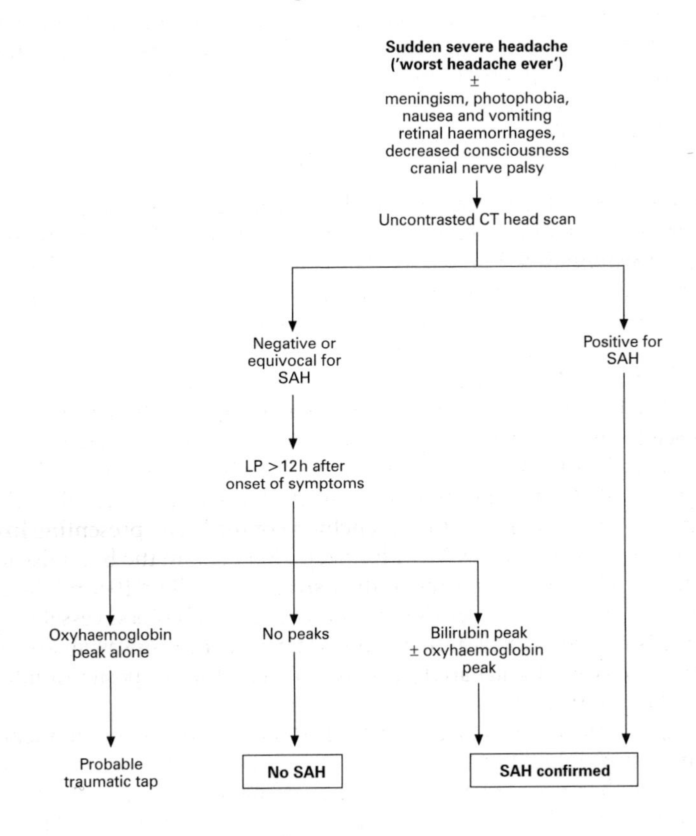

Figure 1. Flow chart demonstrating the decision-making process in the diagnosis of subarachnoid haemorrhage.

Arteriovenous malformations

In an AVM there is a short-circuit between the arterial and venous systems without an intervening capillary system; this leads to a shunt. Patients with these conditions may present with a bleed due to the stresses placed on the fragile venous system, with epilepsy secondary to brain irritation, or with a steal phenomenon (where there is cranial dysfunction of certain parts of the brain which are starved of blood supply because of the short circuit). Around 80% of AVMs will have haemorrhaged by the time the patient has reached the age of 50 years, and there is an increased incidence of bleeding during the third and fourth decades. AVMs are classified according to the Spetzler-Martin (SM) grading system, which has a 1–5 grading. Points are given for size, eloquence of brain and the depth of the draining veins. The size is subdivided into lesions smaller than 3 mm, between 3 and 6 mm, and larger than 6 mm. Location depends on whether the lesion is in an eloquent area (motor/speech area, visual cortex, etc.), and the venous draining system depends on whether it drains superficially or into the central deep veins of the brain. A maximum of 3 points will be given for size, and an extra point added for eloquence or deep-draining vein, giving a maximum score of 5. Small AVMs less than 2 mm can be treated with radiotherapy, but these lesions can take several years before they completely obliterate. Lesions larger than 2 mm that are located superficially in non-eloquent brain can be treated surgically. Other lesions can be treated with a combination of endovascular treatment and surgery, or with endovascular treatment alone. SM grades 4 and 5 are not surgically curable in most instances and it may be safer not to treat.

Cavernous angiomas

Cavernous angiomas are bundles of sinusoidal capillaries which have no arterial supply or venous drainage and have a propensity to bleed. Whereas AVMs can be diagnosed with either conventional, CT, or magnetic resonance angiography, these lesions cannot be demonstrated by angiography, and have to be searched for with conventional MRI scanning. They are thought to be surgically treatable if superficial.

Venous angiomas

Venous angiomas are just coils of veins and can be seen as abnormal areas of veins on angiography and usually do not require any treatment. Venous angiomas, AVMs and cavernous angiomas bleed into the parenchyma and should be searched for in patients who are in their first 6 decades and have had spontaneous bleeds.

Strokes

Strokes can be occlusive or haemorrhagic. Occlusive strokes are due to either venous or arterial occlusion and can have secondary haemorrhagic transformation. Haemorrhagic strokes are usually found in the region of the internal capsule and caudate nuclei where the lenticostriate branches of the middle cerebral artery are found. This is usually because of micro-aneurysms forming on these arteries, secondary to hypertension. Cerebellar hypertensive bleeds are also common, and, less frequently, hypertensive bleeds can be seen in other areas in the different lobes of the brain (lobar hypertensive haemorrhage). Strokes usually occur in older people and are in deep inaccessible brain, and therefore are usually not treated with surgery. The exceptions would be patients who have a cerebellar hypertensive bleed, who are deteriorating secondary to hydrocephalus because of obstruction of the fourth ventricle, and in young patients with nondominant hemisphere lobar bleeds which are close to the surface of the brain.

Traumatic bleeds

Trauma can lead to haemorrhage, either because of direct impact or because of the secondary effects of rotation. Very high velocity impact, like being struck by a baseball bat, is dampened quite successfully by the immersion of brain in CSF and leads only to focal damage. This usually manifests as skin lacerations and subepidermal and subgaleal haematomas, or skull fractures which can lead to tears in the arteries on the dura, such as the middle meningeal artery which can, in turn, lead to extradural haematomas. We also sometimes see subdural haematomas following focal impact. Slower impact and rotational movements, like being involved in a car accident or falling down stairs, lead to the brain's being shaken around inside the skull. This leads to diffuse brain injury; in a mild form, it leads to concussion, and in a severe form, it leads to patient's remaining vegetative, secondary to diffuse white matter damage. As the brain gets shaken around, tearing of the axons takes place and, on a microscopic basis, the diagnosis of diffuse axonal injury can be made. There are three grades of diffuse axonal injury (Grade 2 and Grade 3 patients carry a poorer prognosis):

Grade 1. Patients who suffer injury with the appropriate mechanism and have point bleeds through the parenchyma of the brain on CT scanning.

Grade 2. The presence of point bleeds in the parenchyma and point bleeds in the corpus callosum.

Grade 3. Point bleeds in the dorsolateral brainstem.

Patients with acute subdural haematomas usually have a component of diffuse brain injury, and the subdural haematomas usually result from rotational movement and tearing of the bridging veins between the brain and the dura. Patients with extradural haematomas frequently do not have intrinsic brain damage, but become symptomatic because of external compression of the brain, and, if treated promptly, usually carry a good prognosis. In patients with acute subdural haematomas, the bleed is a manifestation of a more serious underlying brain injury, and the response to treatment is variable. In practice, we usually see a mixture of focal and diffuse brain damage. Smaller pin-point contusions are frequently interspersed with larger bleeds in the parenchyma, called haemorrhagic contusions. These are usually found at the tips of the temporal lobes where the brain tissue comes into contact with bone, and also the inferior frontal lobe, as the brain moves over the rough orbital ridges of the cranial floor. Finding subarachnoid and intraventricular blood indicates that there has been a severe diffuse brain injury.

Because subdural haematomas are caused by blood vessel disruption and, in severe cases, parenchymal disruption, it follows that the mechanism of injury leading to diffuse brain injury (and, on a microscopic level, axonal injury) is tailor-made to cause subdural collections. Diffuse brain injury and subdural collections are, therefore, frequently found together, carrying a grim prognosis. Point bleeds may enlarge to become haemorrhagic contusions. Trauma can also lead to intraparenchymal bleeds; these are usually close to the cortex or come to the surface of the brain.

Extradural collections are caused by focal trauma. Due to the fact that the underlying brain is frequently undamaged, they carry a good prognosis if evacuated promptly before brain herniation sets in. Mixed pathology, resulting in both a diffuse injury and a focal injury, is seen, for instance, in cases where a patient's head hits the windscreen during a road traffic accident (RTA), followed by the car rolling and subjecting the patient to rotational movements and diffuse injury. Contact and focal injuries also frequently lead to *coup–contra-coup* type injuries where soft tissue swelling and skull fracture denotes the site of impact clinically and on CT scan, and an intraparenchymal haematoma or haemorrhagic contusion in the opposite part of the brain denotes contact injury which occurred when the accelerating brain came into contact with the skull.

Disorders of CSF flow

CSF is actively produced by the choroid plexus and ependyma and passively absorbed by the arachnoid villi. The ventricular system in the adult contains approximately 150 ml of CSF and approximately 20 ml/h (nearly 0.5 litres per day) is produced. It follows that, if there is no resorption, the intracranial cavity will be rapidly overinflated with CSF. The irreversible consequence of this is death. Overinflation with CSF leads to dilatation of the ventricular system (ventriculomegaly).

Obstructive (noncommunicating) hydrocephalus

Ventriculomegaly due to an obstruction of CSF flow between the ventricles is characterized by some of the ventricles being over inflated whilst the others, being downstream of the obstruction, remain of normal proportion. This type of ventriculomegaly due to an obstruction is called obstructive hydrocephalus or noncommunicating hydrocephalus. Obstructive (noncommunicating) hydrocephalus can be caused by external compression of the ventricular system by bleeds or tumours or by intraventricular obstruction by tumours or bleeds. Obstruction within the body of the lateral ventricles will lead to only a portion of that ventricle being dilated. Obstruction at the foramen of Munroe will cause the whole lateral ventricle to dilate (anterior horns, body, posterior horns, atrium and temporal horns). Obstruction at the level of the third ventricle obstructing both foramina of Munroe will lead to both lateral ventricles becoming dilated, and lesions at the level of the aqueduct will cause dilation of the lateral ventricles as well as the third ventricle, with the fourth ventricle being of normal calibre. In the cases of aqueduct stenosis, the pressure can be relieved by making a small hole in the floor of the third ventricle with an endoscope during a third ventriculostomy. Ventriculoperitoneal shunting is a very successful treatment of obstructive hydrocephalus.

Communicating hydrocephalus

Hydrocephalus can also occur from failure of CSF absorption by the arachnoid villi. The arachnoid villi can be damaged by infection, SAH, high protein states, and increased venous pressure (e.g., sinus thrombosis). Because there is free communication between the ventricles, this type of ventriculomegaly is known as communicating hydrocephalus. Communicating hydrocephalus can frequently be managed by serial lumbar punctures. If the condition does not clear up, shunting may become necessary.

Hydrocephalus is an excellent demonstration of the Monroe–Kelly doctrine which states that, because the cranium is rigid, the three tissues contained (brain, blood and CSF) have an inverse relation to each other, such that an increase in one leads to a decrease or compression of the other two.

Normal pressure hydrocephalus

Normal pressure hydropcephalus is a term used to describe communicating hydrocephalus in the elderly. It is a misnomer, as the intracranial pressure is usually raised intermittently. Young people usually have small ventricles and so diagnosing hydrocephalus is quite easy in them. In older people, it can be quite difficult. As we get older our brain atrophies, and in keeping with the Monroe–Kelly doctrine this creates more space for CSF, since the blood flow, which is the third intracranial component, does not increase. CSF is, therefore, seen to fill the spaces created by the shrinking brain and this translates on a CT scan to large ventricles, or ventriculomegaly, and enlarged sulcal and cisternal spaces. This is a normal state of affairs. When the ventricles enlarge disproportionally to the cisternal and sulcal spaces, this is called ventriculo-sulcal disproportion and points to a high pressure within the ventricular system. The diagnosis is then suggested of communicating hydrocephalus in the setting of relatively normal intracranial pressure, or normal pressure hydrocephalus. The pathology behind this is thought to be a reduced absorption of CSF due to obliteration of subarachnoid spaces and arachnoid villi dysfunction. The key to diagnosis rests on the clinical picture, which consists of Adam's triad of dementia, ataxia and incontinence, as well as the demonstration of a relative increase in CSF pressure of around 20 cm H_2O on LP. The absolute confirmation comes from an improvement in the symptoms (especially gait) following the removal of 30–50 ml of CSF *via* LP. This then confirms that the symptoms of dementia, ataxia and incontinence are not due just to a normal ageing process. It follows, therefore, that if fluid could be permanently drained off *via* a ventriculoperitoneal shunt, a resolution of symptoms might be expected. The principle is that the shunt, having a valve which opens at a certain pressure, would not allow the pressure to rise above that level. The shunt can have either a fixed valve which has a predetermined pressure or a programmable valve which can be adjusted by an external magnet; the second situation allows the valve to be adjusted in the outpatient department to titrate CSF flow, and so obtain the optimum clinical benefit for the patient.

Benign intracranial hypertension

Another type of CSF absorption dysfunction which leads to a rise in intracranial pressure is thought to be caused by increased venous sinus pressure and is called benign intracranial pressure or pseudotumour cerebrii. This is seen predominantly in young, overweight women and is sometimes due to venous sinus thrombosis. There is certainly nothing benign about this intracranial hypertension despite the name. Due to the decreased absorption of CSF there is a general brain swelling and this diffuses down the length of the optic nerve causing venous stasis in the optic nerve and optic nerve swelling. The main complaints are severe high-pressure headaches and peripheral field deficits. There is no ventriculomegaly (hydrocephalus) in these cases and the ventricles are usually slit-like. Once again, the diagnosis is made by demonstrating high pressures in excess of 20 cm H_2O on LP and demonstrating a decrease in symptoms following drainage of 30–50 ml of CSF. Most cases are managed medically with weight loss, diuretics and sometimes steroids. The visual symptoms can sometimes be alleviated by optic nerve fenestrations done by the ophthalmologists. The headaches and the optic symptoms can frequently be improved by CSF diversion by a shunt. Because the ventricles are usually quite small, and therefore difficult to cannulate, these patients usually have a lumboperitoneal shunt put in; this consists of a catheter that runs from the intraspinal space at level L3/4 to the peritoneum, running under the skin of the flank.

Causes of shunt failure

Many patients with hydrocephalus are treated with a shunt. Most commonly these are ventriculoperitoneal shunts. However, the distal catheter may drain to a variety of body cavities. Shunts are mechanical devices and so may malfunction, resulting in the return of symptoms of hydrocephalus. Shunt dysfunction may be due to infection, blockage or mechanical failure.

Blockage due to infection within the first 3 months is usually due to infection with organisms implanted during surgery. *Staphylococcus epidermidis* and *Staphylococcus aureus* are the main culprits with *S. epidermidis* three times more prevalent than *S. aureus*. The predeliction for this organism in shunt infection is due to the fact that it produces a layer of slime under which it hides and which prevents antibiotics and immune cells from entering. That, coupled with the fact that it lives on the skin of both the patient and the theatre staff, makes it the number one suspect. Shunts should be done by senior staff in daylight hours with the minimum staff in theatre, masks should be worn by all present, the shunt should only be handled with instruments and not hands, and contact between the shunt and the patient's skin should be prevented at all times. Shunt infection can present with meningitis-type symptoms (fever, malaise, headache, photophobia, nausea and vomiting), with raised inflammatory markers, or with symptoms of raised intracranial pressure. Patients may have only raised ICP without external signs of sepsis but with elevated inflammatory markers. The only definite proof of shunt infection is a positive gram stain and culture. It is necessary, therefore, to obtain a CSF sample. This can be done either by tapping the reservoir of the shunt or during open revisional surgery for blockage. We need continually to drain CSF, and therefore we need a catheter to drain the ventricle. Leaving the shunt in and giving antibiotics alone is one possible method of treatment if the shunt is not blocked. However, this only has a 20–30% chance of success. In the still-functioning shunt, removing the distal end to let it drain into a drainage bag whilst giving antibiotics is another option. The CSF collected in the bag is tested from time to time; when the CSF clears of organisms for a good 24–48 h the old shunt is removed and replaced with a new one. This appears to be a very successful way of treating infection of a patent shunt system. In the case of shunt blockage, the best option is to remove the shunt and use an external ventricular drain (EVD) draining into a drainage bag to allow the CSF to clear (as in the option above, where the functioning shunt was externalized distally). Another option is to replace the infected, blocked shunt straight away with a new one. Many neurosurgeons find this option less desirable, however, as placing a piece of plastic into an environment with an abundance of organisms puts the new the shunt at high risk of being colonized and infected (remember the slime layer of *S. epidermidis*). A further discussion on the management of shunt problems can be found in Chapter 7, on ward management of neurosurgical patients.

Congenital disorders presenting in adulthood

Aqueduct stenosis

This is an infrequent cause of obstructive hydrocephalus. Aqueduct stenosis due to congenital anatomic abnormality is not as common as aquired aqueductal stenosis due to external compression.

Chiari malformations

Chiari (Arnold–Chiari) malformations are divided into four subtypes: patients with types III or IV usually die shortly following birth, so only types I and II, therefore, will be seen in clinical practice. It is important to note that Chiari malformations are sometimes referred to as hindbrain hernias for reasons that are evident from the following descriptions.

Chiari I

Chiari I is the adult type and usually presents in the 4th decade of life with a mean presentation at 38 years. The deficit is thought to be due to a large foramen magnum, small posterior fossa and possibly perinatal anoxia. The cerebellar tonsils herniate through the foramen magnum and become compressed. On MRI scanning this is seen as tonsils protruding beyond a line drawn from the anterior to the posterior rim of the foramen magnum. Clinically these patients present with cough headaches, myelopathy and tetraspasticity, vertigo, downbeat nystagmus and the symptoms of syringomyelia. The cough headaches are thought to result from CSF being forced past the tonsils into the posterior fossa. This may also be the cause of an associated syringomyelia. In syringomyelia there are cystic spaces within the spinal cord leading to dysfunction of the sensory modalities, especially spinothalamic sensation, as well as motor dysfunction (spastic paresis being the most common abnormality). Treatment consists of an occipital approach and enlarging the bony rim of the foramen magnum as well as incision of the dura, and duraplasty. Some surgeons do not open the dura as they not only feel that doing so may increase the risk of complications, but believe that not doing so does not reduce the success rate of the procedure.

Chiari II

As in Chiari I, the cerebellar tonsils are herniated through the foramen magnum, but in Chiari II the 4th ventricle and medulla have also herniated beyond the line connecting the anterior and posterior rims of the foramen magnum. Chiari II usually presents in infancy with hydrocephalus and respiratory distress (see Chapter 9, on paediatric neurosurgery). It is usually associated with myelomeningocoele.

Intracranial Infection

Introduction of infection into the nervous system can be by several routes. Direct inoculation can occur during penetrating trauma or during surgery (the infected planes can either be extradural, subdural or intraparenchymal, depending on the extent and site of the inoculation). Haematogenous spread may occur from more distant pathology. This is frequently the case in patients with infected granulations on their heart valves, poor dental hygiene, or abscesses at other sites. The usual presentation is that of intracranial abscesses. Direct spread may occur from nearby paraspinal abscesses or infected cranial sinuses. This usually leads to the formation of an extradural or subdural empyema.

Patients with fever accompanied by convulsions should be assumed to have intracranial sepsis until proven otherwise. It is as easy as that. This is a condition with a great morbidity and mortality. Urgent CT scanning with contrast administration is required to demonstrate the infection and, if this is negative, MRI scanning should be considered since this is more sensitive. Aggressive treatment with high dose antibiotics and emergency surgical drainage is indicated. Long-term antibiotics should be administered intravenously for 6 weeks and oral antibiotics continued until all inflammatory markers and imaging have returned to normal. In some cases this may take months. This is especially true for intracranial abscesses since the protective abscess capsule can be resistant to antibiotic penetration. It is important to appreciate that an abscess can take up to 2 weeks to develop a capsule. The earliest stage of intracranial abscess formation consists of a patchy infection of the parenchyma, known as cerebritis.

SPINAL DISORDERS

There is a bewildering variety of pathology that affects the human spine. The main types of spinal pathology in which the neurosurgeon becomes involved include: tumours; degenerative disease; infection; and, more rarely, bleeds. In addition, there are developmental deformities that may require correction. There are various spinal cord syndromes that result from spinal disease, and it will be useful to become familiar with these. These are, therefore, discussed at the end of this section on spinal pathology.

TUMOURS

It is useful to consider the types of malignancy that most commonly occur in the spine according to the various anatomical spaces that they occupy. Extradural tumours are usually metastatic in nature. They are usually centered on the bone of the vertebra (which has a very good blood supply) with intraspinal extradural extension. Intradural tumours are divided into extramedullary and intramedullary tumours. Intradural extramedullary tumours are usually meningiomas or neurofibromas. Intramedullary tumours are either astrocytomas or ependymomas in the majority of cases.

The basis of treating metastatic spinal tumours is, as in the case of brain tumours, palliation. The main aims of surgery would be to decompress the spinal cord in patients with rapidly progressing deficit, and to stabilize the spine in cases of instability. The main treatment for these tumours consists of radiotherapy and this should be commenced as soon as possible once a tissue diagnosis has been obtained (either by open surgical biopsy or needle biopsy). Intradural, extramedullary tumours are well suited to surgical resection and are mostly benign. Intramedullary tumours are also treated with surgery, and ependymomas are usually more benign than the astrocytomas. Radiotherapy is also used as adjuvant therapy.

DEGENERATIVE DISEASE

Neural compromise due to compression is usually due to the bony compression of spinal stenosis or to disc degeneration and prolapse. The areas where the stable segments of the spine (the thoracic and sacral spines) join the more mobile segments of the spine (the cervical and lumbar spines) is where the most stress is placed and disc degeneration and prolapse occurs. The most usual segments for this are C6/7, C5/6 and C7/T1 in the cervical spine, and L4/5 and L5/S1 in the lumbar spine. Thoracic disc disease is more unusual. Patients who present with disc prolapse usually do so in the first four decades of their life and there is usually a precipitating event, such as a fall or picking up a heavy object. The disc is composed of a central soft part, the nucleus pulposus, and a tougher outer fibre layer, the annulus fibrosis. Damage to the annular fibres leads to damaged disc material herniating through into the spinal canal. There are various ways in which the separate stages of disc prolapse can be described. In our opinion, the following four terms provide a useful descriptive classification.

1. *Disc bulge:* annular damage with the disc material bulging but still contained by the annular fibres.
2. *Disc protrusion:* the disc fragments protrude through the annular fibres.
3. *Disc extrusion:* the disc material has completely migrated outside the anatomical boundaries of the disc space. On an MRI scan this is seen as a fragment bulging into the spinal canal.
4. *Sequestered fragment:* a piece of disc has broken off and lies loose within the canal.

The single all-encompassing term for the above is *disc prolapse*. The usual initial symptom from disc prolapse is back pain followed by radicular (nerve root) pain. Radicular pain is pain that is caused by nerve root compression and the pain manifests in the dermatome supplied by that specific nerve root.

It is important to understand the anatomy of the spine and the relation of the nerves to the surrounding structures, and to tie that in with the anatomy of the dermatomes. The nerve root of a corresponding segment leaves under the pedicle of the vertebra of that segment. Thus the L5 nerve root leaves under the pedicle of L5 which is opposite the L5/S1 disc space. The nerve root of L5 thus lies quite lateral in the anatomical area opposite the L5/S1 disc space and will be compressed by a disc prolapse which is off the midline in the lateral recess and neural foramen. A disc prolapse in the midline will compress the S1 nerve root on its way to the nerve root foramen under the pedicle of S1. Therefore, at any one given level, a lateral disc will compress the nerve root of that level, whilst a central disc herniation will compress the nerve root of the level below. Compression of a nerve root leads to numbness and paraesthesia, pain and muscle weakness. We can work out from the sensory symptoms and the dermatomes which nerve root is being compressed. The other diagnostic tool is myotome dysfunction: e.g., a central L4/5 (compression of L5 nerve root) disc prolapse will lead to weakness of ankle dorsiflexion and toe dorsiflexion, whereas a L5/S1 disc prolapse (compression of S1 nerve root) will lead to weakness of ankle eversion and plantar flexion with a dropped ankle reflex.

Cervical disc disease causes neck pain, radicular symptoms and myelopathy. Because of the presence of spinal cord in the cervical area (rather than nerve roots as in the lumbar region), central disc herniations will compress the cord and lead to a myelopathy with spasticity in all four limbs. A lateral disc will compress the nerve root and lead to radicular symptoms with pain, numbness and paraesthesia and weakness. A broad central disc can cause both a myelopathy and a radiculopathy, and patients are said to have a radiculomyelopathy. We can once again identify the level according to the dermatomes and myotomes. Spinal stenosis is a disease of general wear and tear and usually occurs from the 5th decade onwards. In the cervical area this leads to slowly progressive myelopathy and sometimes to acute paresis following a sudden extension injury, such as a fall following a slip in the bathroom. The critical diameter of the cervical cord is about 13 mm and compression beyond that leads to symptoms of myelopathy and weakness.

Spinal stenosis in the lumbar area leads to claudication. Unlike arterial claudication, which can occur at rest, neurogenic claudication usually follows walking, and, in severe cases, just standing. The pain is in the calf and is relieved by flexing the hips and standing bent over or sitting down. This leads to less strain on the nerve roots and usually relieves the pain. Spinal claudication is therefore posture related and the pulses are readily palpable, denoting an adequate vascularity. Spinal stenosis is thought to begin with disc degeneration, leading to excess mobility. This is thought to lead, in turn, to facet joint hypertrophy and ligamentum flavum hypertrophy, with resultant auto bony fusion, as the body tries to negate this mobility. Eventually, there is a decrease in spinal canal diameter and the patient becomes symptomatic due to compression of the neural structures. Spinal stenosis is treated surgically by decompressive laminectomy. Surgery for a disc prolapse is in the form of a discectomy. However, it is important not to forget that conservative management of disc prolapse can be very successful. Discectomies can be *via* a number of approaches, including microdiscectomies (*via* a small bony opening of only a part of the lamina), hemilaminectomies, full laminectomies, or *via* lateral approaches to the exit foramina for laterally placed disc prolapses.

INFECTION

Infection of the spine follows the same basic pathological principles as in the brain, and three mechanisms – metastatic spread, direct extension and direct inoculation – are responsible for infection. Metastatic cancer spreads to the vertebral bodies, whereas metastatic infection spreads to the disc space causing discitis with severe local back pain, pressure tenderness over the affected segment, fever, and raised white cell count and inflammatory markers. Discitis frequently leads to extradural empyema with compression of the thecal sac and the spinal cord contained within the upper spine and the cauda equina contained in the lower part of the lumbar canal. These patients are not only toxic, but also have neurological deficits. Extradural empyema is a feared complication of epidural anaesthesia, and discitis can follow discectomy. Treatment of discitis involves strict bed rest and a long course of IV antibiotics (usually >6 weeks). Extradural empyema requires emergency surgical drainage, followed by bed rest and antibiotics.

SPINAL CORD SYNDROMES

It is helpful to split these syndromes according to whether they occur in the upper or lower parts of the spinal canal.

Syndromes of the upper spinal cord

Anterior spinal cord syndrome

This is due to dysfunction of the cord tissue supplied by the anterior spinal artery and can follow occlusion or damage to this artery, or it is due to anterior compression. It is manifested by muscle weakness below the level of the injury as the motor fibres have an anterior course in the spine. Usually, soft touch (carried anteriorly) and pain and temperature sensation (carried laterally) are also involved. This is an extensive lesion with usually only proprioception (carried posteriorly) intact, and carries a poor prognosis.

Central cord syndrome

This is usually due to hyperextension injury in the elderly where an already critically narrowed diameter of a spinal canal leads to cord compression. The motor fibres in the spinal cord are arranged with the lowest fibres – the legs – being outermost and the fibres of the arms being innermost. A central cord syndrome therefore damages the inner fibres more than the outer fibres, leading to arm weakness that is greater than leg weakness. There is usually a variable amount of sensory deficit as well.

Bell's cruciate paralysis

This is seen in victims of trauma who have intact function of their legs but weakness in their arms. This is because the arm fibres cross higher in the spine than do the leg fibres, and a focal injury of the central spinal cord at the point of decussation leads to this phenomenon.

Syndromes of the lower spinal cord

Remember that, in the lower part of the lumbar canal, beyond the conus, there are only nerve roots (cauda equina).

Conus medullaris syndrome

This is due to compression of the conus, which is at L1/2 level. This is the origin of the cauda equina, and compression leads to both spinal cord compression (myelopathy with spastic weakness and sensory deficits) and nerve root compression (radiculopathy with pain, paraesthasia and lower motor neurone flaccid weakness as well as sphincter disturbance).

Cauda equina syndrome

This is frequently seen as a neurosurgical emergency due to sphincter dysfunction. Compression of the roots leads to the usual radicular symptoms of pain, paraesthesia and weakness, but the more sinister component is the compression of the sacral nerve roots that supply perianal, perineal, rectal and bladder sensation as well as sphincter control of both the bladder and the rectum, and erectile function in males. Emergency surgery to remove the compressive element is needed within 24 h of the onset of urinary incontinence/retention or rectal incontinence to save sphincter function. Saddle anaesthesia is usually a warning symptom of pending catastrophe.

PERIPHERAL NERVE DISORDERS

Peripheral nervous system pathology is predominantly the territory of the neurologist. However, there are various peripheral nerve compression syndromes that are amenable to treatment by neurosurgeons.

Compression of the median nerve under the flexor retinaculum leads to pain in the median distribution, as well as to paraesthesia. This is known as carpal tunnel syndrome. Patients frequently awake from sleep with a severely painful hand which improves with elevation. The history is distinctive and tapping over the flexor retinaculum can elicit the symptoms in severe cases (Tinnel's sign), as can holding the wrist fully flexed for >60 s (Phalen's sign). The diagnosis is confirmed with electromyography (EMG) studies and surgical treatment includes carpal tunnel decompression (see the section on basic surgical procedures).

Ulnar nerve compression can occur in the forearm at the wrist (Guyon's canal) or at the elbow, leading to pain, paraesthesia and paralysis in the ulnar distribution. Surgical release can be quite successful, e.g., ulnar nerve transposition at the elbow.

Peripheral nerve dysfunction may also be caused by peripheral nerve or nerve sheath tumours.

4

Neurosurgical History and Examination

CONTENTS

INTRODUCTION

Taking a good history and performing a competent neurosurgical examination requires a basic level of knowledge and understanding of the various types of neurosurgical pathology. It is for this reason that this chapter follows the preceding overview of neurosurgical pathology. You should endeavour to use the history and examination to produce a fairly reliable working diagnosis and to localize pathology. Bear in mind non-neurosurgical pathology (e.g., acutely ischaemic legs can mimic a cauda equina lesion), so make sure to enquire about vascular symptoms and feel (and document!) for relevant pulses. The history and examination discussed here are focussed on patients who are alert enough to be on the ward.

HISTORY

This is the most important of all. Listen carefully and allow patients sufficient time to speak. There is no such thing as a 'poor historian' – rather it is a reflection of a lack of skill on our part as history-takers. Have a diagnosis in mind when you have finished, or at least a differential diagnosis; otherwise ask more probing questions to help yourself. Be able to verify which part of the nervous system the pathology is most likely to be located in, and roughly what type of disease process you are expecting. For instance, in the patient who has difficulty walking, it is important to appreciate, and to differentiate between, spinal and cranial pathology, and equally important to distinguish between the different types of pathology – vascular, degenerative, oncological, etc. Be sure to find out, therefore, whether the history is progressive or of sudden onset. You should by now have some appreciation of the significance of different types of headache, e.g., early morning headaches (raised intracranial pressure), sudden onset occipital headache (SAH), cough- or strain-related occipital headache (hindbrain hernia). Relevant associated symptoms should be inquired about, e.g., fevers, photophobia, alterations in vision, urinary and faecal continence. Be sure to ask about relevant risk factors and associations, e.g., in patients with SAH ask about smoking, family history, polycystic kidney disease.

EXAMINATION

THE AWAKE PATIENT

This is by no means a comprehensive and detailed overview of the intricacies of neurological examination. It attempts, however, to give broad guidelines and background that would be useful in everyday practice. Being pleasant and open in your approach helps patients to settle down quickly and be more compliant. It is very important always to have a system. There are several approaches, and the following is a comfortable one.

Mental function and orientation

A quick assessment can be made by asking patients a series of questions about themselves and their surroundings. The questions below constitute the abbreviated mental test score (AMT score) which is given out of 10 (1 point for each question). A common mistake is to refer to this as the mini-mental state examination (MMSE). However, the MMSE takes longer to do, includes drawing tests and is scored out of 30.

1. What is your age?
2. What time is it (to the nearest hour)?
3. Can you remember this address – 42 West Street (recall at end of test)?
4. What year is it?
5. Where are you now (name of hospital)?
6. Can you tell me who these people are or what they do (recognition of two people, e.g., a nurse, a doctor)?
7. What is your date of birth?
8. What year did World War I start?
9. Can you name the present monarch?
10. Can you count backwards from 20 to 1 in threes?

Cranial nerve function

CN I

The olfactory nerve is rarely dysfunctional, except in cases of subfrontal tumours, like meningiomas, or in trauma with an anterior skull-base fracture. Smell function can be tested with a pinch of coffee, each nostril being examined separately whilst pinching the opposite nostril. Intact olfactory function can more conveniently be verified by asking the patient whether they can smell their food.

CN II

We are mostly interested in compression and the dysfunction resulting from it. The optic nerves run in close proximity to the carotid artery and the cavernous sinus, as they extend backwards to the chiasm in front of the lamina terminalis, which is the anterior margin of the 3rd ventricle. From there, they pass around the brain stem to the lateral geniculate body, from where the optic radiations emerge, going to the calcarine cortex in the occipital lobes.

The visual pathways and the defects produced by various lesions in the pathways are summarized in Figure 2. Images are transmitted from the retina backwards *via* the optic nerves, with the nasal fibres crossing over and the temporal fibres continuing straight backwards. The lower retinal fibres cross anteriorly (upper temporal visual field) and the upper retinal fibres cross posteriorly in the chiasm (lower temporal field). As the fibres reach the lateral geniculate body, the fibres fan out in an optic radiation, the fibres serving the lower nasal retina (upper temporal field) dipping into the temporal

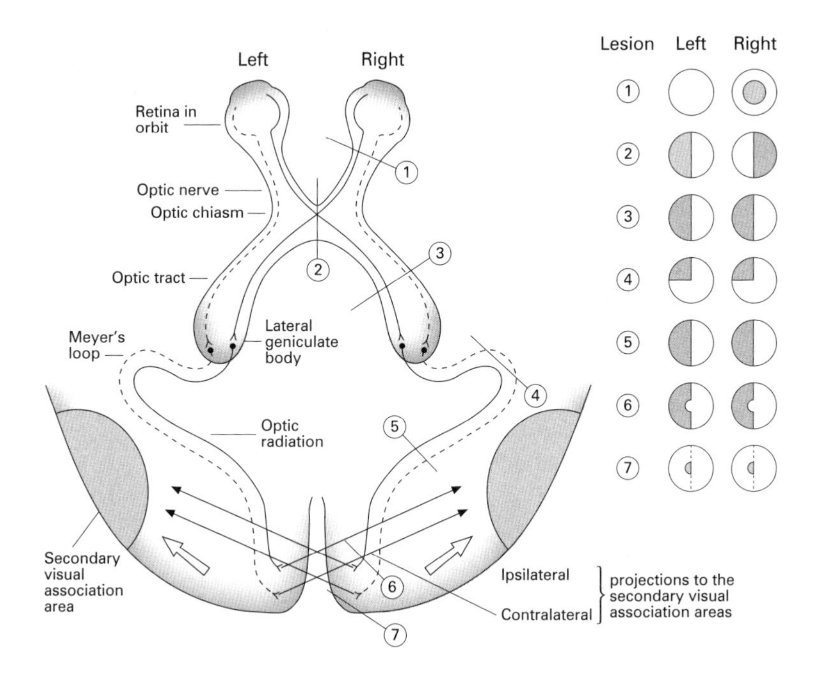

Figure 2. Diagrammatic representation of the visual pathways from the retina to the cerebral cortex. The visual deficits shown are due to the lesions indicated: (1) right optic nerve; (2) optic chiasm; (3) right optic tract; (4) right Meyer's loop; (5) right optic radiation; (6) right calcarine cortex; (7) tip of right occipital lobe. Note that the outer part of the visual field may be spared in an early compressive lesion of the optic nerve. The secondary projections to the ipsilateral and contralateral visual association areas are also shown (note that the contralateral projection is much weaker). These are important to understanding the basis of attention hemianopia. If there is a lesion in the right parietal visual association area (serving the left visual field) the contralateral (left parietal) area will allow vision, provided that there is no concomitant input to the left side from the right visual field. This reflects the weakness of the secondary contralateral projections compared to the ipsilateral inputs to the visual association areas. Clinically, attention hemianopia is demonstrated by asking the patient to identify two fingers moving in each side of the visual fields. If the patient can identify fingers moving in one side of the field when they are moved alone but not when fingers in both sides are moved, then they have an attention hemianopia.

lobe: this part of the optic radiation is known as Meyer's loop. It thus follows that a lesion in the left temporal lobe will cause a deficit in the information carried by the fibres originating on the right nasal retina (upper temporal field). The fibres originating in the left lower temporal retina on the left-hand side also pass through Meyer's loop and a lesion here therefore results in a right-sided upper quadrant homonymous hemianopia. The fibres then reach the calcarine cortex of the occipital lobe where images are recorded, and we become aware of them as the occipital cortex has relays to the visual association areas in the parietal lobes bilaterally. The contralateral relay is much weaker than the ipsilateral relay and this is the basis for inattention hemianopia. Although a lesion in the right parietal lobe means the patient should not have awareness of an image recorded in the occipital lobe, the patient is nevertheless aware of the image because of contralateral relay to the opposite visual association area. If, however, at the same time, there is an image in the right visual field, which will relay to the left occipital cortex, the ipsilateral input to the left visual association area will obliterate the weaker contralateral input from the right occipital area and the patient will no longer see the image in the left visual field (see Figure 2). We can demonstrate this in practice by testing visual awareness with a finger placed in the contralateral visual field to where the lesion is, and showing that introducing a finger into the ipsilateral visual field to where the lesion is, causes the patient no longer to see the initial finger.

Understanding the basics of the visual relay helps us to locate a lesion accurately from visual confrontation. This is done by sitting opposite to the patient with your eyes at the same level as theirs; you then ask the patient to block off their right eye with their right hand while you block off your left eye with your left hand. Then, starting on the left-hand side, you bring your finger (or a red pin) in from the periphery and you note the position in which the patient detects your finger (or the pin). The reason for using a red pin is that an inability to see red is the first deficiency that appears with optic nerve compression. This procedure, known as the confrontation test, is done in superior, lateral, inferior and medial peripheries of one eye and then repeated with the other eye, with the patient similarly occluding their eye. This easily demonstrates any field deficit that might be present. Remember to document the visual fields as the patient would see them. The presence of intact vision and full visual fields indicates a free flow of information along the optic nerves. Any deficit, therefore, is a sign of compression or obstruction to the flow of this information.

The four typical lesions that we find are:

- A lesion of a single optic nerve before it reaches the chiasm: this will result in loss of vision in a single eye Therefore, a compression, or loss of function, of the left optic nerve will result in left eye blindness.
- A lesion compressing the chiasm: this will initially compress only the nasal fibres which cross over, because the temporal fibres, which do not cross over, are more laterally situated. This lesion will lead to a loss of vision in both temporal visual fields.
- A lesion in the temporal lobe: this will, as described previously, lead to a contralateral upper quadrant homonymous hemianopia.

- A lesion in the parietal or occipital cortex: this will lead to a contralateral homonymous hemianopia of both the upper and the lower quadrants.

Assessing visual acuity is also an intrinsic part of testing the function of the optic nerve, although people can have near complete obliteration of their optic field and still have intact visual acuity. Visual acuity is tested with an eye chart at a distance of 6 m. The vision is documented as a fraction of 1; a value of 1 indicates normal vision, i.e., an ability to read the 6 m line with the chart placed at 6 m (denoting the ability to see the same size letters as a person with normal vision would be able to see at 6 m). The patient with the worst recordable vision would be one who could see at 6 m only letters of a size that a person with normal vision would be able to see at 60 m; therefore it is recorded as one tenth of normal vision, or 6/60.

The third and last step of testing the optic nerve is by doing fundoscopy. It is, perhaps, the case that never have more lies been told in medicine than in the reporting of fundoscopic results. There is frequently general confusion about fundoscopy, and the skill to diagnose papilloedema comes only with repeated examinations of different normal fundi. The term papilloedema means bilateral disc swelling and should be reserved for that. It is best to note down whether optic disc swelling is left-sided or right-sided. Papilloedema takes 10–14 days to develop, and is thus unlikely to be present in acute neurosurgical pathology. It is therefore important to realize that lumbar puncture in a patient with intracranial pathology might be hazardous, even though the fundoscopy is normal. There are four very easy-to-remember stages in the development of papilloedema.

Stage 1. The back pressure in the optic nerve leads to decreased ability of the veins to drain, and therefore there is an increase in venous calibre and tortuosity. It is also possible, with experience, to see a decreased venous pulsation.

Stage 2. Because of the swelling, the optic disc changes from its normal pale colour to pink, and starts to swell, causing the vessels that usually plunge into the disc to stop abruptly at its margins.

Stage 3. The disc margins have now become indistinct and blurred.

Stage 4. The disc now is elevated, pink and swollen, and it is quite common to see haemorrhages around the veins.

Fundoscopy is useful, therefore, for detecting papilloedema that is usually present in cases of long-standing tumours or hydrocephalus, but it is also useful for detecting haemorrhages. In SAH we do see – albeit infrequently – retinal and vitreous haemorrhages (Terson's syndrome) and subhyaloid haemorrhages (bleeding beneath the subarachnoid membrane).

CN III, IV, VI

Examination of the oculomotor nerve has two components. The third cranial nerve works together as a team with the second cranial nerve to constrict the pupil, and works together with the fourth and sixth cranial nerves to move the eye around in the orbit. A light-stimulated impulse travels back in the optic nerve to reach the lateral geniculate body; then, in the brain stem at the level of the superior colliculus, fibres are given off bilaterally to the Edinger-Westphal nuclei. From the Edinger-Westphal nuclei a parasympathetic pathway passes through the brainstem, quite close by an area called the conversion centre, into the third cranial nerves of both sides. Both the Edinger-Westphal nuclei and both oculomotor nerves are thus activated by input from a single side, and we therefore have a bilateral, consensual reaction to a unilateral input (see Figure 3). As the impulse travels down the oculomotor nerves, it reaches the ciliary ganglion from where the short ciliary nerves serve the sphincter pupillae to cause a pupillary constriction. The

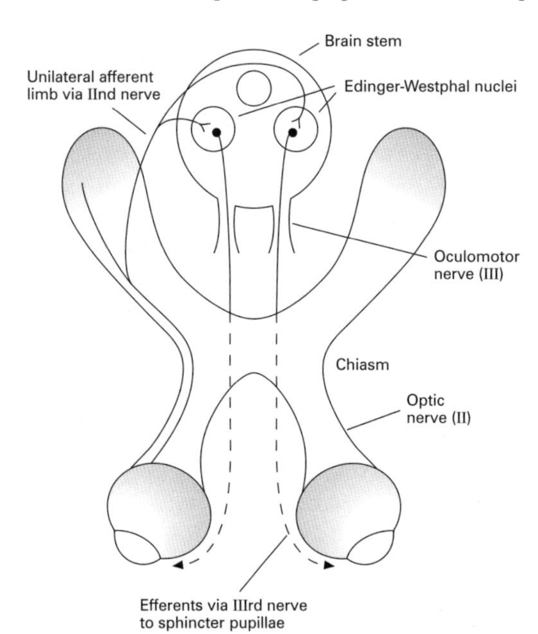

Figure 3. Diagrammatic representation of the afferent and efferent limbs of the pupillary reflex. Note that the afferent limb conveys impulses from a single eye to both Edinger-Westphal nuclei. This is the basis of the consensual light reflex where light shone into one eye causes bilateral pupillary constriction.

fibres of the oculomotor nerve that mediate sphincter constriction lie on the surface of the nerve on the dorsal aspect and are, therefore, usually involved quite early on in compression of the third nerve. Pupil constriction is therefore a parasympathetic function, mediated by the third nerve following activation of a parasympathetic nucleus by the second cranial nerve. Damage to the afferent pathway (retina, optic nerve, chiasm and optic tract) leads to a pupillary response known as the Marcus Gunn pupil. This is elicited by swinging a flashlight in a pendulum motion between the two pupils. As the light falls on the unaffected eye, both pupils will constrict fully because of the afferent input on both Edinger-Westphal nuclei. As the light falls onto the affected eye, the affected pupil will, instead of constricting, slightly dilate because of the decrease of afferent input due to afferent pathway damage. Efferent pathway lesions lead to a loss of constriction and therefore to dilatation of the pupil served by the oculomotor nerve, which denotes dysfunction caused either by intrinsic mechanisms or by extrinsic compression. The fact that the pupillo-constrictor fibres lie superficially on the third nerve is an important distinguishing factor between medical dysfunction of the third nerve and a surgical (compressive) lesion. Third nerve dysfunction where there is involvement of the pupil is usually compressive. The third nerve also carries some sympathetic fibres which innervate the superior and inferior tarsus muscles of Muller which assist eye opening. The first component of a third nerve compression is therefore dilatation of the pupil, and the second is ptosis.

Pupillary dilatation is brought about by sympathetic activity, which is initiated in the hypothalamus and then descends down into the spinal cord to the level of T1. At the level of T1, the white rami of the nerve roots of C8 and T1 pass to the cervical sympathetic ganglion and from here sympathetic nerves enter the cranial cavity on the surface of the carotid artery, and are delivered to the pupil *via* a branch of the ophthalmic nerve. Dysfunction of this system leads to ptosis (because of decreased supply to the tarsus muscles), myosis (loss of mydriasis) and anhydrosis (loss of sweating) – the so-called Horner's syndrome.

The second main function of the third cranial nerve is movement of the eyeball, in conjunction with the fourth and sixth cranial nerves. The third cranial nerve supplies all the muscles of the eyeball, except for the superior oblique and lateral rectus muscles: this can be remembered easily using the formula, $(LR_6 SO_4)3$. A patient with a full third nerve palsy will, as we have discussed before, have a dilatation of the pupil, as well as a ptosis. They will also have a pupil which is looking downwards and outwards. This is because of the unopposed pull of the lateral rectus and superior oblique muscles. The lateral rectus muscle causes the eyeball to look towards the outside, and the superior oblique muscle, which hooks around a trochlea, causes the eye to look inferiorly. It follows that lateral rectus palsy causes an inability of the affected eye to look laterally. It is difficult (and quite rare) to find an isolated fourth nerve palsy: when it does occur, it usually presents with diplopia on looking outward and downward because of superior oblique dysfunction. This can best be conceptualized by recalling that the superior oblique pulls the eye down and medially, whilst the inferior rectus pulls the eye down and laterally. In a patient with a fourth cranial nerve palsy, downward gaze results in the unopposed action of the inferior rectus pulling the affected eye down and out. Downward gaze, therefore, precipitates or worsens diplopia.

CN V

The three branches of the trigeminal nerve traverse the cranial cavity in three separate places: the mandibular nerve enters through the foramen ovale; the maxillary nerve enters through the foramen rotundum; and the ophthalmic division through the superior orbital fissure. The trigeminal nerve is mostly sensory and supplies sensation to the whole face. The mandibular nerve carries the motor part and this supplies the muscles of mastication. Examination of the trigeminal nerve primarily tests the sensation of the first, second and third division, as well as the corneal reflex (which is part of the first division). Power of muscles of mastication, as well as the jaw jerk, which are part of the evaluation of the trigeminal nerve, are of lesser clinical significance.

It is important to recall that the third, fourth, and sixth cranial nerves, as well as the first division of the trigeminal nerve, run through the cavernous sinus and can be compromized by lesions there. Patients with intracavernous aneurysms, tumours, or arteriovenous fistulae, frequently have palsies of the third, fourth and sixth cranial nerves, and of the first division of the trigeminal nerve on the ipsilateral side.

CN VII

The facial nerve is almost purely motor and supplies all the muscles involved in facial expression. It also has a sensory component to the external auditory canal and conveys taste from the anterior two thirds of the tongue *via* the chorda tympani. Clinical evaluation of the seventh cranial nerve hinges on the understanding that there are two separate components to facial nerve function: the first is the supranuclear innervation of the muscles of facial expression, and the second is mainly concerned with reflex eye closure and does not have a cortical component. Both eyes will shut if there is any danger to either individual eye, and therefore there is dual innervation of both sides of the forehead. This leads to the finding of intact upper face function in patients who have had a hemispheric incident, such as a stroke.

The fifth, seventh and eighth cranial nerves are located in a space between the pons of the brain stem, the cerebellum, and the cranial base, in an area called the cerebellopontine angle.

CN VIII

The vestibulocochlear nerve really consists of two nerves, with the cochlear nerve relaying hearing from the cochlea, and the vestibular nerve relaying information from the apparatus of balance (the semicircular canals and otolith organs). Acute events, such as trauma and infection, cause decreased hearing as well as balance problems. Chronic compression leads to a decrease in hearing, though balance remains intact due to compensation by the contralateral vestibular function. Hearing can be crudely tested by rubbing your fingers together at the side of the patient's ear and determining whether the patient can hear the movement. Webber and Rinne testing can be extremely useful to distinguish between conductive and sensorineural deafness. If more information is needed about hearing function, a patient should be referred to an audiologist.

CN IX, X, XI

The ninth, tenth and eleventh cranial nerves are usually tested together. The reason for this is anatomical. These three nerves share the same motor nucleus, the nucleus ambiguus, in the medulla (although the accessory also has a spinal nucleus) and they all exit the skull by the same route (through the jugular foramen). This close anatomical association within the confines of the skull means that is unusual for centrally located pathology to produce isolated lesions of these cranial nerves.

The glossopharyngeal nerve (IX) is the main afferent path of the gag reflex, supplies some sensation around the external auditory canal, and conveys taste from the posterior third of the tongue. The only clinically significant aspect is the afferent part of the gag reflex. The vagus nerve (X) also helps to convey sensation from the ear but is the main afferent pathway for the gag reflex. The vagus nerve is also motor to most of the muscles of the palate. Testing the ninth and tenth cranial nerves thus consists of testing the gag reflex, which demonstrates an intact afferent pathway (ninth cranial nerve) and efferent pathway (tenth cranial nerve) and also testing palatal function by asking a patient to open their mouth and say 'aah'. If there is a palsy, the muscles that are intact on the unaffected side will pull the palate in that direction and therefore demonstrate the palsy.

The spinal accessory nerve (XI) originates in a nucleus in the spinal cord, leaves the spinal cord through cervical branches, and then goes on to supply the sternocleidomastoid and trapezius muscles on the ipsilateral side. This nerve is unusual in that the higher control is not crossed and a right-sided lesion will therefore lead to a right-sided nerve dysfunction. The function of the eleventh nerve is tested by asking the patient to lift the ipsilateral shoulder up against resistance to test power in the trapezius muscle: the patient is then asked to turn his head away from the side being tested whilst pressure is applied to the head while the patient is looking in the contralateral direction, and the sternocleidomastoid muscle is palpated to check for a good muscle action and bulk. A right sternocleidomastoid and right eleventh nerve function is therefore tested by asking the patient to look towards the left against resistance and palpating the muscle on the right-hand side.

CN XII

The hypoglossal nerve (XII) supplies the motor fibres of the tongue and is tested by asking the patient to open their mouth and let the tongue lie loosely in the mouth. Fasciculations are noted at this point, and the patient is then asked to stick his tongue out and move it from side to side. If there is a palsy, the stronger and intact side will push the tongue over towards the weak side.

Cranial nerve testing

It is extremely important to develop a quick and efficient manner of testing the cranial nerves. Usually the first cranial nerve is not tested, except when there is a clinical suspicion; the second cranial nerve is tested by doing acuity visual confrontation fields and fundoscopy; the third, fourth and sixth cranial nerves are tested together by checking the movements of the eye; the fifth cranial nerve is checked by noting the sensation in the face; the seventh cranial nerve is tested by asking the patient to move their face in a grimace, to whistle, and to wrinkle their forehead; the eighth cranial nerve is tested by rubbing your fingers together close to the patient's ear; and the lower cranial nerves are testing by examining the gag reflex, looking at palatal function, checking shoulder and neck movements, and finally by looking at movements of the tongue. If practised, this can be done quickly and in sequence within a few minutes.

After noting down the history and asking a few pointed questions to ascertain the patient's mental function, and when the cranial nerves are fully tested, it is time to move on to the rest of the neurological examination.

Motor system

As we know, motor function is controlled contralaterally in the cerebral hemisphere, and there can be dysfunction anywhere from the motor cortex, corona radiata, internal capsule, the decussation in the medulla, to the spinal cord and peripheral nerves. These are the so-called pyramidal pathways. Motor function is also dependent on the extrapyramidal system, and upon the modulation supplied by the cerebellum. Table 1 summarizes myotomes and dermatomes. Even minor dysfunction can be demonstrated by forcing a patient to rely on both the pyramidal system (intact power) and extrapyramidal system (positional feedback and proprioception). This can be done by asking a patient to hold their arms outstretched in front of them and asking them to make a piano-playing movement in the air. Alternatively, you can ask them to close their eyes and stand with their arms outstretched, palms facing up. Inability to do piano-playing movements, or a drift towards the inside (pronator drift), indicates mild weakness. This is useful for testing patients who have cranial dysfunction. Power is noted on a scale of 1–5, with 5 being normal power, 4 being mildly reduced power, 3 indicating anti-gravity power, 2 indicating movement which is not able to defy gravity, and 1 indicating a flicker. The MRC scale is summarized in Chapter 13 (Table 6), on scoring systems in neurosurgery.

The pyramidal system

Trying to decide the location of the dysfunction causing a power deficit can be confusing, but if we stick to a few simple rules it should be fairly obvious. If there is abnormal power, there has to be a dysfunction at some point between the brain and the muscle. In neurosurgery, we do not usually

Table 1. Summary of myotomes, dermatomes and root values of common reflexes.

Nerve root	Myotome (muscles supplied)	Action	Reflex	Dermatome
C5	Deltoid Biceps	Shoulder abduction Elbow flexion	Biceps jerk	Lateral forearm
C6	Biceps Brachioradialis	Elbow flexion Elbow flexion	Biceps jerk Brachio-radialis jerk	Thumb
C7	Triceps	Elbow extension	Triceps jerk	Middle finger
C8	Flexors digitorum	Finger flexion	–	Little finger
T1	Intrinsic nuscles of the hand	Finger abduction and adduction	–	Medial forearm
L1	Hip flexors	Hip flexion	–	Anterior thigh & inguinal area
L2	Hip flexors	Hip flexion	–	Anterior thigh
L3	Quadriceps	Knee extension	Knee jerk	Anterior thigh
L4	Quadriceps	Knee extension	Knee jerk	Anteriormedial thigh
	Tibialis anterior	Ankle dorsiflexion and foot inversion	–	–
L5	Extensor hallucis longus	Big toe extension	–	Lateral leg
S1	Ankle	Plantar flexion	Ankle jerk	Posterior lower leg and lateral side of foot
S2	Ankle	Plantar flexion		

get to deal with muscle abnormalities, and will therefore ignore those. Lesions of the brain pathways or the spinal cord will cause weakness, but will also decrease the higher modulation of reflex activity in the spinal cord. This will cause patients to have overactive reflexes and therefore to appear spastic. It is important to realize that the lower part of the lumbar spine does not contain spinal cord, but only the cauda equina, and so only lesions above the level of L1/2 will lead to spasticity; a lesion from L3 downwards cannot lead to spasticity. Above L3, the rule that governs the level of dysfunction is different. At the level of the lesion you may find lower motor neurone signs, and therefore weakness without spasticity (decreased reflex), whilst at the level below that you will find weakness with increased reflexes and spasticity. Thus, a cord lesion at C5 will lead to decreased power in the biceps and reduction in the brachioradialis reflex, but spastic reflexes in the fingers and in the lower limbs.

The basis for finding the origin of weakness is the absence or presence or spasticity and the level of that spasticity. For instance, a patient with compression in the thoracic cord will have spastic legs, but normal tone and reflexes in the arms; a patient with compression of the brain or the cervical cord will have both spastic arms and legs. Patients with lumbar disc disease can never be spastic due to their disc. A patient with both facial weakness and a hemiparesis obviously has a cranial dysfunction and needs a CT scan of his brain.

Reflexes should be noted as absent, present with reinforcement, present, increased, increased with nonsustained clonus, or increased with clonus.

Extrapyramidal system

The cerebellum is the main modulator of movement, and integrates proprioceptive feedback from all over the body to modify and change motor signals to our muscles. As a general rule, lesions of the cerbellar vermis will lead to truncal ataxia and an inability to stay upright whilst sitting in bed. Hemispheric cerebellar lesions tend to cause ipsilateral limb ataxia. A left cerebellar lesion thus causes ataxia in the left arm and left leg.

A patient with cerebellar disease will usually be hypotonic on the side of the lesion, reflexes will be decreased, and nystagmus is common. Limb ataxia in the upper limbs can be elicited by asking a patient to touch their nose and then to touch your finger which is held about 60 cm or so away from the patient's nose; the movement is then repeated rapidly to and fro. The patient will frequently not be able to touch your finger, and will point past it. There will also be a shaky and unsteady movement of the hand. It is also not possible for the patient to keep their hands outstretched and do piano playing movements (this will already have been picked up in the screening test for motor dysfunction). The lower limbs can be tested for ataxia by asking the patient to run the heel of one foot up and down the shin of the other leg, starting at the knee and returning to it. This will usually be a very shaky and uncoordinated movement if there is ataxia present. The final test to confirm the ataxia is to ask the patient to do rapid and alternating movements, such as tapping his foot on the floor or tapping the back of one hand with the other hand as fast as he can. An inability to do this is termed dysdiadochokinesis.

Evaluation of gait is an often neglected but important part of neurological examination. Patients with severe lower back and radicular pain will have an antalgic type of gait where they put less pressure on the affected side. In patients with cerebellar disease, there is a general unsteadiness due to limb ataxia. In patients with a CVA, there is usually fixed flexion of the upper limb and a straight, outstretched leg with plantar flexed foot, which causes them to walk by circumducting the affected leg (swinging the stiff, outstretched leg out and around before placing it down). Patients who are myelopathic have a stiff and spastic gait and frequently shuffle along.

It is, therefore, quite obvious that a lot can be learned from observing a patient's gait. Romberg's test depends on our need for at least two out of three senses (proprioception, middle ear, vision) to be able to stand unaided. Therefore, closing the eyes will cause patients to fall over backwards or forwards if they have either middle ear pathology or decreased proprioception. As can be imagined, this is not a very specific test, and has little clinical value.

Sensory system

When testing sensation, you basically have to test four modalities: light touch, pain, temperature and joint position sense.

Light touch is tested by lightly touching the patient's skin, either with your finger tips or with cotton wool, down the whole length of the body and comparing results between each side of the body.

Pain sensation is tested with pin-prick and this is usually quite successful in delineating sensory level. It is important to compare normal with abnormal and also to compare the two sides of the body. If you think that a patient has a sensory lesion at the T4 level, it is useful to compare sensation in the face with sensation on the trunk; sensation on the face would probably be normal. Be careful not to fall into the 'C4–T4 trap': these dermatomes are very close on the trunk and it is possible to misdiagnose a C4 lesion as a T4 lesion. We then also have to compare left to right. It is usually unnecessary also to test temperature sensation, since the two modalities, pain and temperature, are closely related physiologically (fibres for both modalities run together in the spinothalamic tracts).

Two-point discrimination is reliable only when tested on the fingertips where discrimination of 3–5 mm should be sensed by a normal patient. Joint position sense should be tested in both hands and both feet, and is quite a reliable indicator of abnormal function of the sensory cortex. There is no specific clinical significance in testing vibration sense.

When testing sensation, we really want either to indicate a level at which sensation changes or ends, or to show a hemispherically-located decrease in recorded sensation, when comparing the two sides. Sensation testing is an aid in localizing pathology and is discussed further in the chapter on spinal disease.

THE COMATOSE PATIENT

Competent assessment of the comatose patient requires accurate assessment of the Glasgow Coma Scale (GCS) score and searching for focal deficits by evaluating pupillary responses and motor function.

Glasgow Coma Scale

The GCS is an excellent tool. Unfortunately, there are too many people who do not fully understand it and seem frightened to use it. Being awake does not equate to a GCS of 15/15, and being difficult to rouse does not mean that the patient is confused. The GCS score is a very biological measurement; it is not a measure of a patient's alertness, so much as of their ability to defend and look after themself. This can be seen when the three components of the GCS are considered in turn.

The motor response

This is prognostically the most valuable part of the GCS. A full mark is 6/6 and the worst mark is 1/6.

6/6 being able to follow commands which need a rather sophisticated train of events in the nervous system;
5/6 aware of, and being able to localize, a painful stimulus (pain) in order to defend oneself (called purposeful flexion or localizing to pain);
4/6 aware of, and flexing to, but unable to find, the threatening stimulus (reported as non-purposeful flexion);
3/6 decortication, when the arms are spasmodically fully flexed next to the body (this can be thought of as an action that has no reliance on the cognition of the cortex – decortication);
2/6 decerebration, when the arms are spasmodically extended on either side of the body, the legs also are spastic and extended (think of a stage of spinal reflex that does not rely on the cerebrum at all – decerebration); this and the previous stage are called posturing, and have a grim prognosis;
1/6 no motor response.

Speech

A full mark is 5/5. This can sometimes be misleading, as a lesion in the speech area might be small, but sufficient to cause a person to lose speech and thus lead to a score of only 1/5 in the speech component, thereby dropping the total GCS total score to 11/15.

5/5 fully orientated person to place, time and person (orientation);
4/5 confused speech without full orientation (confusion);
3/5 words;
2/5 sounds;
1/5 no sounds.

Eye opening

A full mark would be 4/4 and the lowest mark 1/4. Being able to see a threat is crucial to an organism's ability to defend itself.

4/4 spontaneously has eyes open;
3/4 will open eyes to speech or sound and is aware of surroundings;
2/4 so unresponsive that only a painful stimulus is enough to make the patient aware of a threat, and is unaware of surroundings;
1/4 no stimulus is enough to make the patient open his/her eyes.

Total score

The total GCS score is 15. The lowest GCS is 3/15 and this is true in patients who are fully sedated, those who are only functioning on their brainstem or those who have even lost this primal function and who are thus brain dead. See the section on ICU management to see how to test for brainstem function.

Focal deficits

Pupillary function

Pupillary dilatation is a symptom of herniation and increased ICP and it is an important warning sign. This is tested as one of the brainstem reflexes.

Motor function

It is important to establish whether there is a hemiparesis (weakness) or hemiplegia (no function). A comatose or confused patient's examination is usually restricted to the GCS, pupillary response, and presence or absence of a paresis.

5

Interpretation of CT Head Scans

CONTENTS

Infections (cerebritis and abscess)
Cortical injury
    Diffuse axonal injury
    Cortical contusions
Infarction
Some common cysts
    Arachnoid cyst
    Colloid cyst

INTRODUCTION

Identifying neurosurgical abnormalities on CT head scans need be no more difficult than interpreting a chest X-ray. Similar principles apply.

Confirm the patient details and date of the scan. This also helps you to put the scan up correctly since to read the patients details you have to have the scan the right way up and not back-to-front. Identify whether the scan is with or without contrast. Work through the scan in an ordered and systematic fashion. If there is an obvious abnormality, describe all its features, i.e., site, shape, density and homogeneity, and whether or not it enhances. Ensure that you go back and check all your review areas to make sure you don't miss anything. To be able to do all these things, you need to have a system of working through the scan, and to know how to identify the gross anatomical structures on a CT scan so that you can localize the lesion. You will also need to know the terms that are used to describe cranial CT lesions. It will be useful to have a simple mnemonic to ensure you have checked everything.

CRANIAL ANATOMY ON CT SCAN

You need to able to identify the following areas: spaces (ventricular system, cisterns); parenchyma (lobes of hemispheres, cerebellum, brainstem, basal ganglia); dural folds (tentorium, falx); sinuses (sagittal sinus). Figure 4 shows the main features of a normal axial CT head scan.

DESCRIBING LESIONS

Describing lesions is very important. You should be able to describe a scan over the phone to a senior colleague. It is essential to use a system and terms that everyone is familiar with and understands. The following features of a lesion should be covered when describing them on scans.

- *Site*: anatomy (see above); is the lesion intrinsic (within the parenchyma) or extrinsic (arising outwith the parenchyma, but may be pushing into it)?
- *Shape*: diffuse or well-circumscribed; smooth or irregular edge.

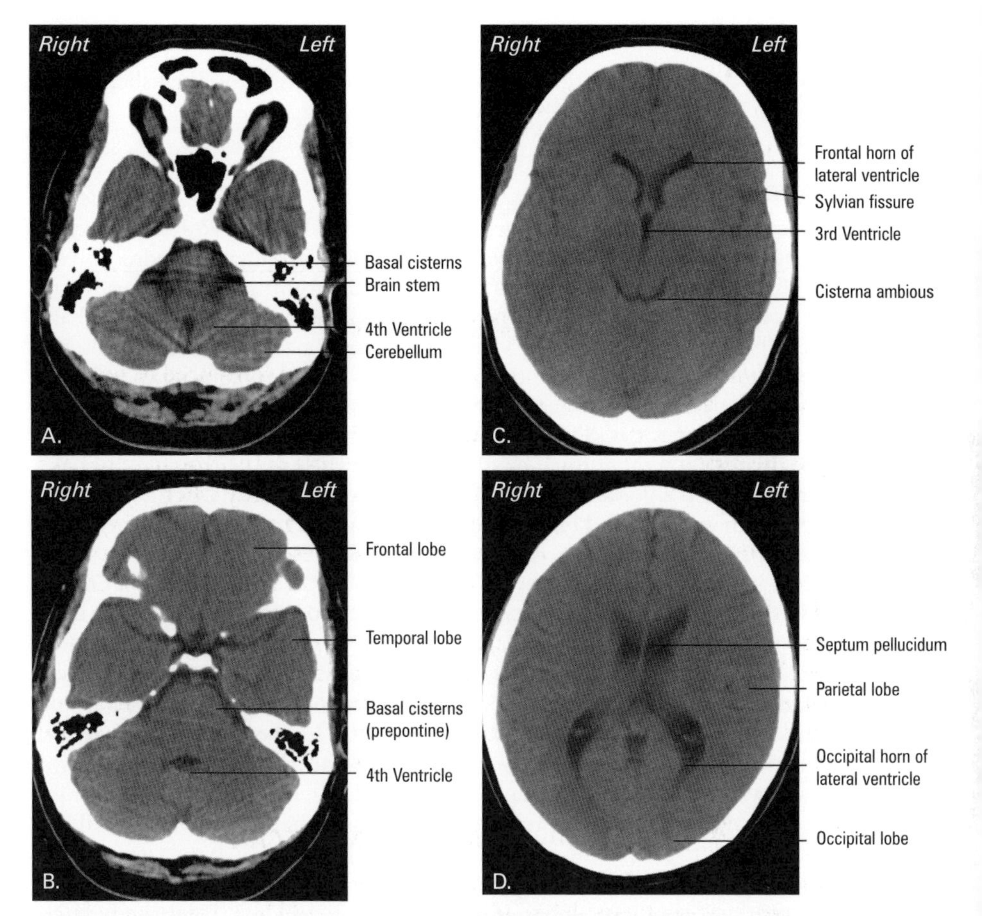

Figure 4. Features of a series of normal axial CT head scans from caudal (A) to rostral (D). The key features that should be identifiable on a CT head scan are annotated. Note that the location of the right and left side of the patient reflects the radiological convention of looking at scans from a caudal viewpoint.

- *Density*: hyperdense (whiter than brain), hypodense (darker than brain), or isodense (same density as brain).
- *Homogeneity*: homogeneous or inhomogeneous density.
- *Enhancement*: enhancing (regularly, irregularly or ring-enhancing) or non-enhancing; the significance of enhancement is that it indicates that the blood–brain barrier has been breached, or that there is neovascularity.
- *Associated features*: e.g., surrounding oedema, dural origin, calcification.

A SYSTEM OF REVIEW

Start at the bottom of the head and work up through the axial slices.

CSF SPACES

Ventricular system

The ventricular system comprises the 4th ventricle, the aqueduct, the 3rd ventricle, and the lateral ventricles. The aim here is to identify hydrocephalus and, if it is present, to determine whether it is communicating or obstructive. Note in particular the temporal horns (see Figures 13, 15, 16, 23 and 25). These are not normally visible in younger people and their presence indicates that there is hydrocephalus. Once hydrocephalus has been identified, see whether there is any obvious level of obstruction. For example, if the 4th ventricle is of normal size but the ventricles above (3rd and lateral) are dilated then there must be obstruction at the level of the aqueduct. See Figure 16 for a good example of obstructive hydrocephalus due to blood in the 4th ventricle and Figure 25 for an example of hydrocephalus secondary to obstruction at the level of the 3rd ventricle.

Basal cisterns

Reviewing the basal cisterns is particularly important as it can help in determining whether or not intervention is required. For example, if an elderly man with a small chronic subdural haematoma has no midline shift and his basal cisterns are widely open, then he may not require intervention as he has room to compensate for the mass effect of the haematoma. On the other hand, if the basal cisterns are completely obliterated in a diffuse head injury then it may be that intervention will not alter the outcome as the patient has already coned. The basal cisterns also communicate with the subarachnoid space and are therefore one of the commonest sites in which to identify subarachnoid blood (see the features of SAH, below).

SYMMETRY OF BRAIN SUBSTANCE AND TISSUES

Work up from the foramen magnum through the cerebellum, basal ganglia and internal/external capsule to the hemispheres. Look for any symmetry, as any asymmetry indicates that something is wrong somewhere. If there is shift to one side, examine the contralateral side carefully for any space-occupying lesions. Look in particular at the sulci and sylvian fissures. They may be effaced if there is a compressive lesion. It is useful to look at the skull and the extracranial tissues as any asymmetry due to fractures or scalp swelling can give clues to the presence of intracranial lesions. If anything abnormal is seen, try to identify which part of the brain it is in. Does the location of the lesion conform to the history? A useful tip is that if you can see the falx in the midline, then you are above the tentorium.

CONSISTENCY OF SCAN AND HISTORY

It is essential to confirm that the scan is consistent with the history. For example, a patient with a history of a gradual-onset, right-sided weakness and a scan showing a small, right-sided, acute, basal ganglia bleed does not add up. In this case it would be necessary to look for left-sided pathology, such as infarct or subdural haematoma, or it might be necessary to consider spinal pathology. Also, a scan might look horrendous but the patient might actually be better clinically. In this case, ensure that you have the correct patient's scans and check the date of the scans. Consider carefully the sequence of events. For example, consider a patient who fell off their bike and has subarachnoid blood on the scan. Did they have a spontaneous bleed from an aneursym and then fall off their bike, or were they knocked off by a car, in which case they may have had a traumatic bleed?

A CHECK-LIST MNEMONIC

The following mnemonic (CT SCAN) provides a useful check-list to ensure that you haven't missed anything.

C	CSF flow: ventricular system
T	Tissues: symmetry of intracranial, cranial and extracranial tissues
S	Sulci and sylvian fissures
C	Cisterns
A	Abnormal blood: look for SAH, epidural haemorrhage (EDH), subdural haemorrhage (SDH)
N	Never forget the history! Is the scan consistent with the history?

CT FEATURES OF COMMON NEUROSURGICAL CONDITIONS

To formulate a differential diagnosis you need to know the features typical of common neurosurgical conditions. These conditions have characteristic patterns in terms of site, shape, density, homogeneity, enhancement, and any additional features. It was pointed out earlier that, in very broad terms, neurosurgical pathology can be divided into haemorrhage and tumours. It is useful, therefore, to consider typical CT features of common conditions under these headings. In addition, we will consider CT features of other neurosurgical conditions, namely abscesses, diffuse head injury, common cysts, and infarction.

HAEMORRHAGE

It is useful to remember the different appearances of extravasated blood on CT scans. Acute blood (<72 h) is hyperdense (white), subacute blood (72 h to 1 week) is isodense, and chronic blood (>1 week) is hypodense.

Traumatic bleeds

Extradural haematoma (see Figures 5 and 6)

- Between skull and brain.
- Biconvex (inner convexity pushing into brain) due to the fact that the dura is being stripped away from the bone.
- Hyperdense.

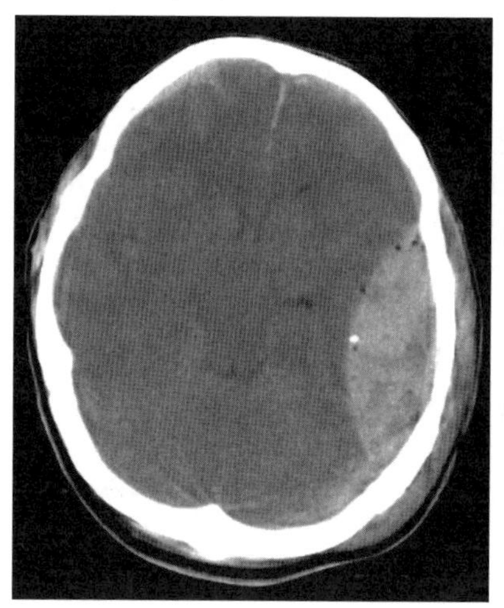

Figure 5. Axial CT head scan showing a large, left-sided, parietofrontal extradural haematoma. Note that the haematoma is biconvex and hyperdense. This haematoma is probably due to rupture of the left middle meningeal artery. There are also some hyperdense areas at the frontal poles that may represent contusions from a *contra-coup* injury. The presence of extracranial soft-tissue swelling on the left side is further evidence that the blow is likely to have been to the left side of the head.

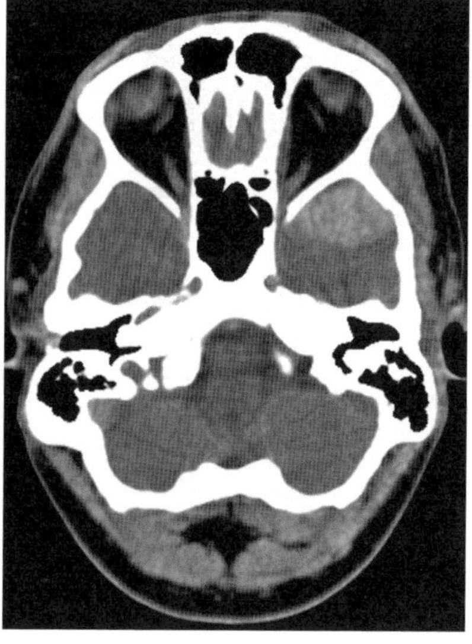

Figure 6. Axial CT head scan showing a left-sided temporal haematoma. Note the classic crescentic shape and hyperdense appearance.

Subdural haematoma (see Figures 7–12)

- Between skull and brain.
- Crescentic (follows contour of brain).
- Hyperdense (acute), isodense (subacute), or hypodense (chronic).
- Loculation and membranes may be visible in chronic subdural haematomas (CSDH).

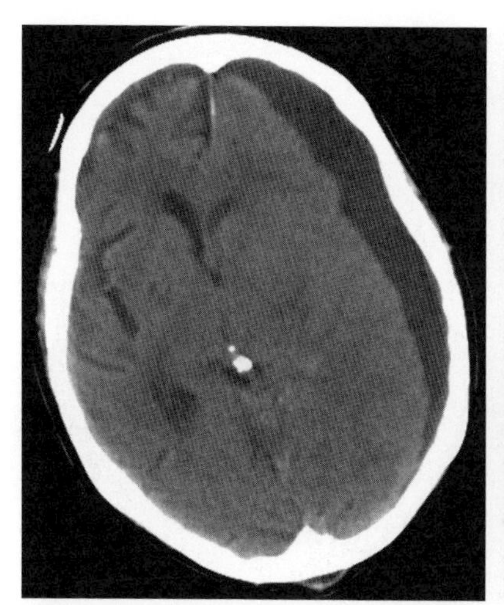

Figure 7. Axial CT head scan showing a large, left-sided, chronic subdural haematoma covering the convexity of the whole hemisphere. There is significant midline shift (>1cm) with distortion of the ventricular system. The haematoma is crescentic and hypodense. Note that the sulci over the left hemisphere have been effaced. In smaller haematomas this may be the only sign indicating the presence of subdural blood, especially if the blood is subacute and isodense (see Figure 9).

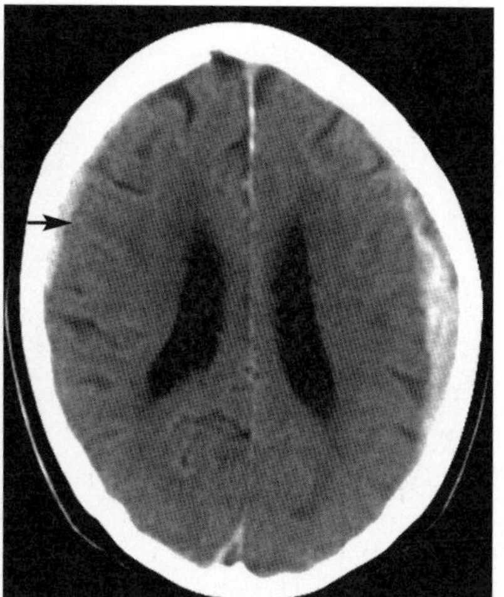

Figure 8. Axial CT head scan showing a left-sided, frontoparietal, acute subdural haematoma. The haematoma is crescentic and hyperdense. Note that there is also some acute subdural blood on the right side (arrow).

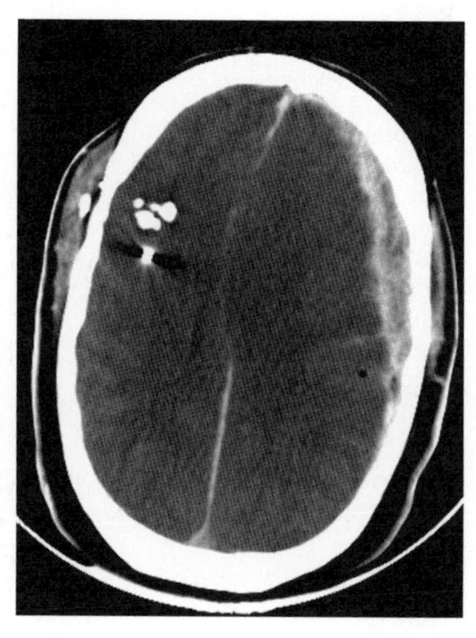

Figure 9. Axial CT scan showing a left-sided, frontoparietal, subdural haematoma (crescentic and hyperdense). Note that there are also some hyperdense areas in the right hemisphere with some associated scatter effect. This is usually seen with radio-opaque foreign material. There are also a couple of hypodense areas within the parenchyma suggesting the presence of intracranial air. Swollen parenchyma is also contributing to the shift to the right side Unfortunately, this patient was shot at close range through the head with a low calibre weapon. The foreign bodies in the right hemisphere are the remnant of the bullet and/or fragments of bone.

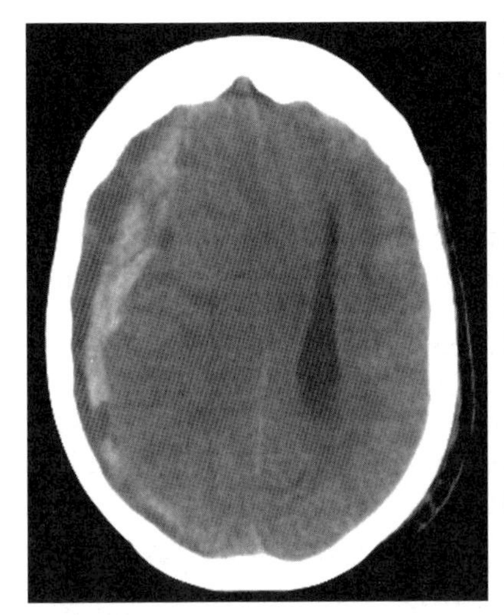

Figure 10. Axial CT head scan showing a right-sided, acute-on-chronic, subdural haematoma covering most of the right hemisphere. Note the crescentic shape and the mixture of hypodense and hyperdense areas indicating, respectively, old and new blood.

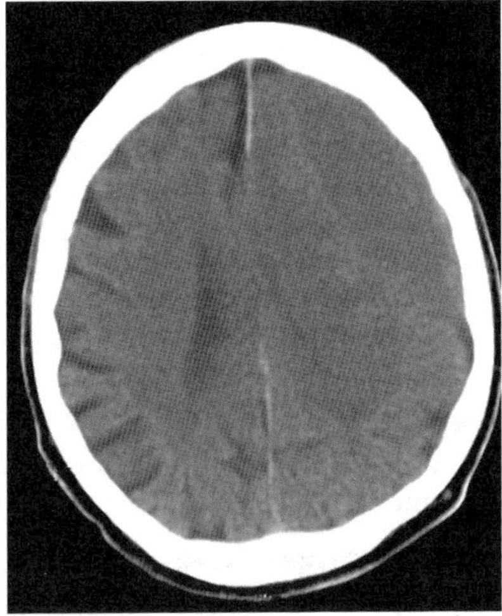

Figure 11. Axial CT head scan showing a large, subacute, left-sided, subdural haematoma. The haematoma is beginning to turn hypodense. However, the clear asymmetry seen in the scan is more evident because of the absence of obvious sulci in the left hemisphere.

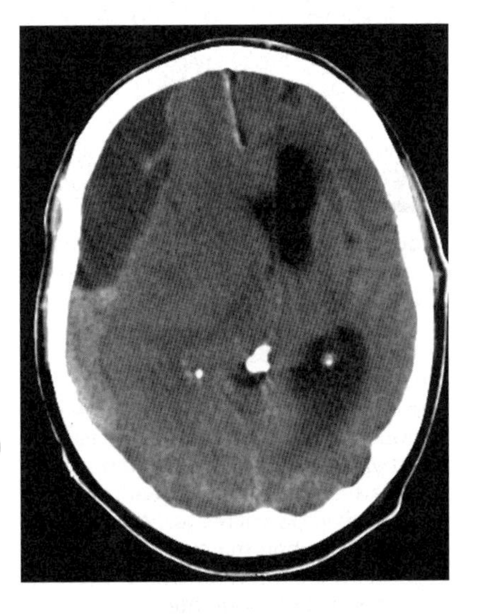

Figure 12. Axial CT head scan showing a large, right-sided, chronic, subdural haematoma with massive midline shift. Note that there is a horizontal level demarcating the upper hypodense area from a lower hyperdense area. It is possible that the hyperdense area represents a further acute bleed separated by membranes from the chronic component. However, it is more likely that this is simply sedimentation of an old bleed.

Spontaneous bleeds

Subarachnoid haemorrhage (see Figures 13–17)

- Subarachnoid space
  - Basal cisterns: circle of Willis aneurysms
  - Sylvian fissure: internal carotid, posterior communicating artery (Pcomm), or middle cerebral artery (MCA) aneurysms
  - Interhemispheric fissure and anterior flame-shaped intraparenchymal haemorrhage: anterior communicating artery (Acomm) aneurysm (the most common aneurysm).
- Diffuse streaks following surface of brain.
- Hyperintense – but after 1 week may not be visible due to dissipation by CSF flow. (CT scans are 98% sensitive in the first 12 h for SAH, but sensitivity declines to 70% by day 3).

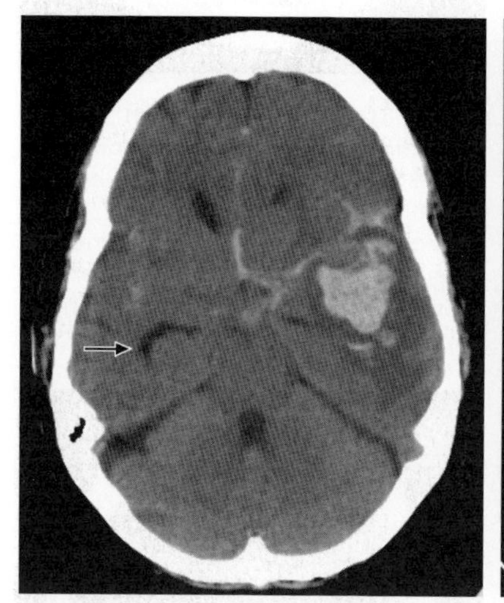

Figure 13. Axial CT head scan showing the presence of acute subarachnoid blood. There is also a large left temporal intraparenchymal haematoma (hyperdense). Interestingly, the middle cerebral artery aneurysm responsible for this bleed can be seen silhouetted against this haematoma. The hypodense area around the haematoma reflects the swelling in the surrounding parenchyma. The other noteworthy abnormality is the enlarged right temporal horn (arrow) indicating the presence of moderate hydrocephalus.

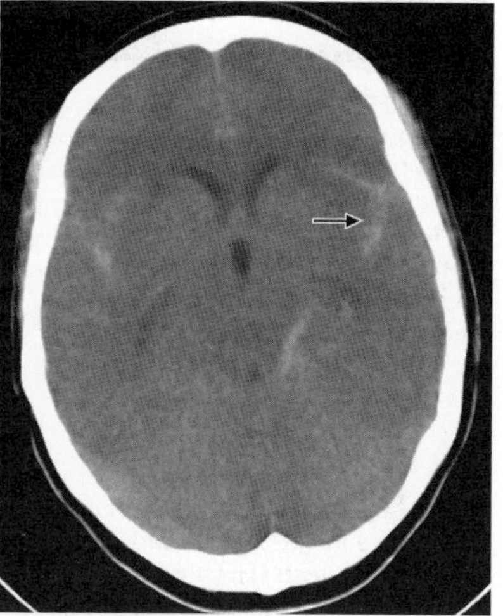

Figure 14. Axial CT head scan showing the presence of subarachnoid blood (hyperdense). Note in particular the presence of blood in the left sylvian fissure (arrow).

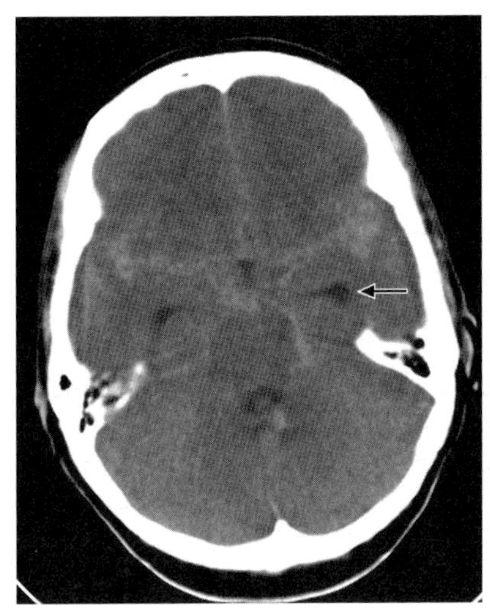

Figure 15. Axial CT head scan showing diffuse subarachnoid blood (hyperdense). Note that the temporal horns are slightly enlarged, indicating the presence of hydrocephalus (arrow indicates left temporal horn).

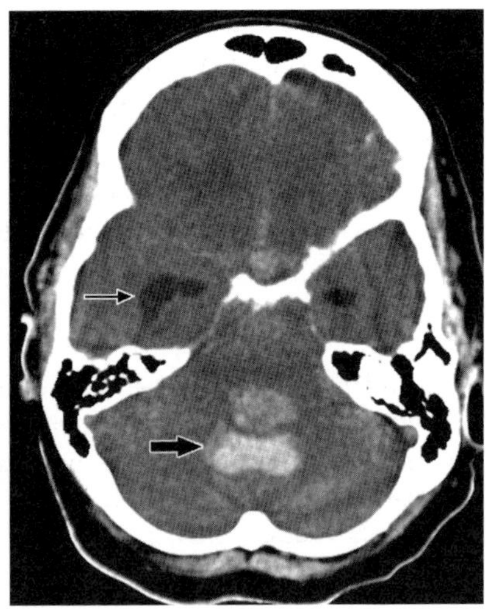

Figure 16. Axial CT head scan showing the presence of subarachnoid blood and a large collection of blood in the 4th ventricle (thick arrow). This obstruction of the 4th ventricle is causing hydrocephalus, as evidenced by the enlarged temporal horns on this scan (thin arrow).

Figure 17. Axial CT head scan showing a large, intraventricular bleed. Blood can be seen in the 3rd ventricle (thick arrow) and frontal horns of the lateral ventricles (thin arrow). The presence of ventriculomegaly confirms the presence of obstructive hydrocephalus.

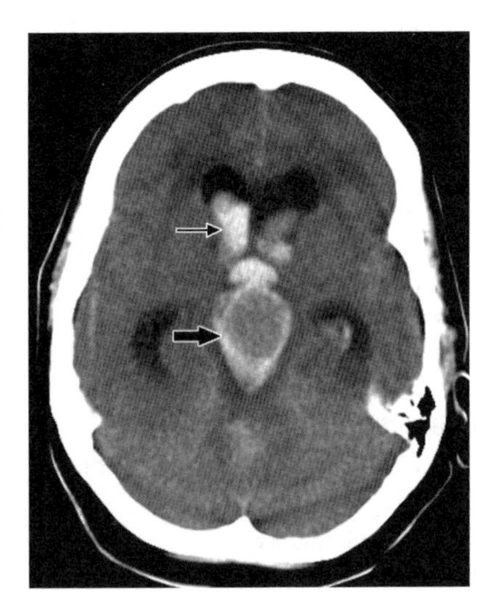

Hypertensive bleeds

- Most commonly basal ganglia and cerebellum, but can be a lobar intraparenchymal cerebral bleed.
- Vary in shape.
- Hyperdense in acute phase.
- Hypodense area may surround clot due to oedema.
- Usually elderly hypertensive patient, but not exclusively so.

AVM

- Similar features to hypertensive bleed but more cortical location and more likely to occur in normotensive younger patients.
- Frequently have an underlying 'salt and pepper' appearance with the mass of underlying vessels faintly visible on an uncontrasted scan and vividly visible following the administration of contrast.

TUMOURS

Metastases (see Figure 18)

- Intraparenchymal (intrinsic) and may be multiple.
- Well-circumscribed.
- Mixed density.
- Inhomogeneous.
- Enhancing: either inhomogeneously or ring-enhancing and can have central necrotic areas.

Gliomas

Low-grade (see Figure 19)

- Intraparenchymal (intrinsic).
- Regular shape but poorly defined edges.
- Hypo- or isodense.
- Homogeneous.
- Non-enhancing (except for juvenile pilocytic astrocytoma).

High grade (see Figure 20)

- Intraparenchymal (intrinsic).
- Irregular and may be diffuse.
- Mixed density.
- Inhomogeneous.
- Strongly enhancing (in an inhomogeneous fashion) with central necrosis in the highest grade – glioblastoma multiforme (GBM).

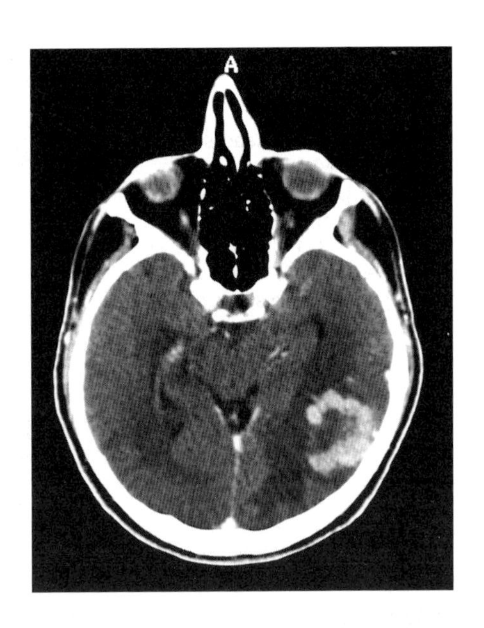

Figure 18. Axial CT head scan with contrast, showing a metastasis in the left parietal lobe. Note that the lesion is well-circumscribed, enhancing, and of mixed density. There is probably some central necrosis.

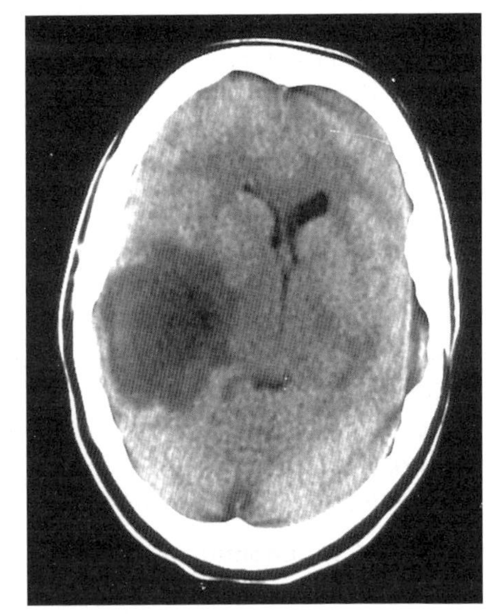

Figure 19. Axial CT head scan of a large, low grade glioma of the right parietal lobe. The lesion is hypodense and virtually homogeneous.

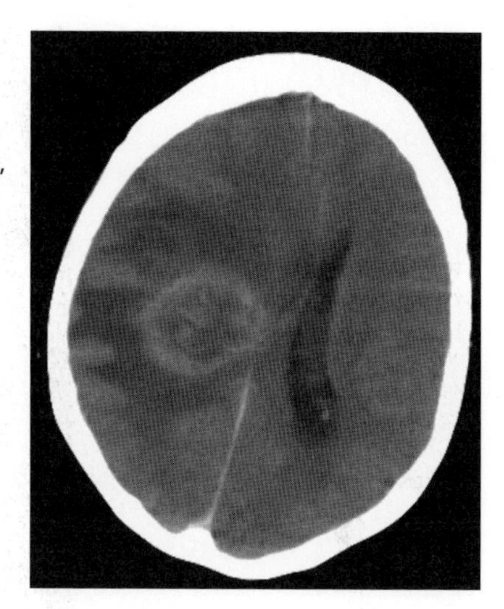

Figure 20. Axial CT head scan with contrast, showing a large, right-sided, enhancing, parietal space-occupying lesion with surrounding oedema (hypodense area) and midline shift. The centre of the lesion is inhomogeneous. This is a high grade glioma with a necrotic centre.

Meningiomas (see Figure 21)

- Extrinsic – although appearing parenchymal they will always have a dural origin.
- Well-circumscribed smooth or lobular.
- Hyperdense.
- Homogeneous.
- Enhance homogeneously (they light up like a light bulb).
- Skull changes – associated with skull erosion and thought to be a malignant feature. Other meningiomas are associated with hyperostosis, much like fibrous dysplasia.

Oligodendrogliomas (see Figure 22)

- Most often in the frontal lobes but can appear anywhere, including the intraventricular space.
- Calcification is almost invariably present.
- Inhomogeneous appearance.
- Inhomogeneous enhancement.

Primary CNS lymphomas

- Periventricular intraparenchymal (intrinsic).
- Irregular.
- Hyperdense with surrounding hypodensity (oedema).
- Homogeneous.
- Enhance homogeneously.
- Disappear with steroids ('ghost tumours').

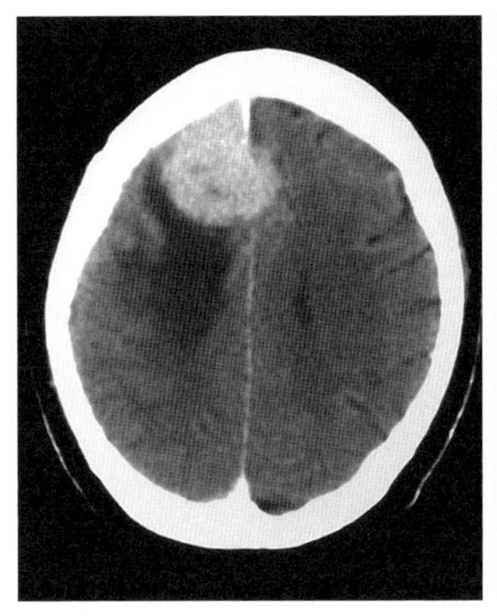

Figure 21. Axial CT head scan with contrast, showing a right frontal meningioma. The lesion is enhancing and homogeneous with a dural attachment.

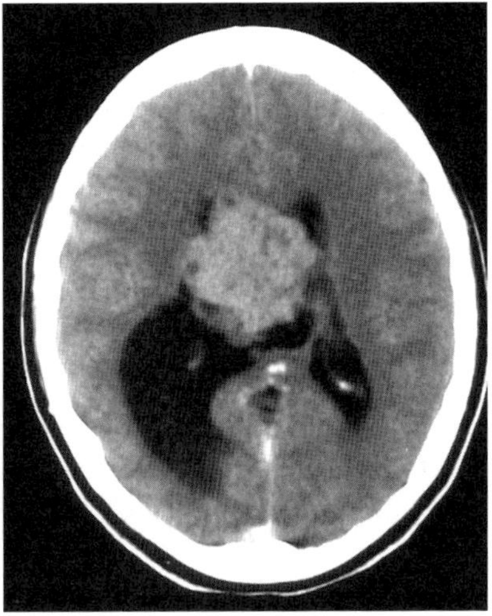

Figure 22. Axial CT head scan with contrast, showing an inhomogeneous, intraventricular oligodendroglioma.

Figure 23. Axial CT head scan with contrast, showing a ring-enhancing, cystic, space-occupying lesion in the posterior fossa (cerebellum). Note the effacement of the 4th ventricle and the presence of obstructive hydrocephalus as evidenced by distended temporal horns. This is a haemangioblastoma.

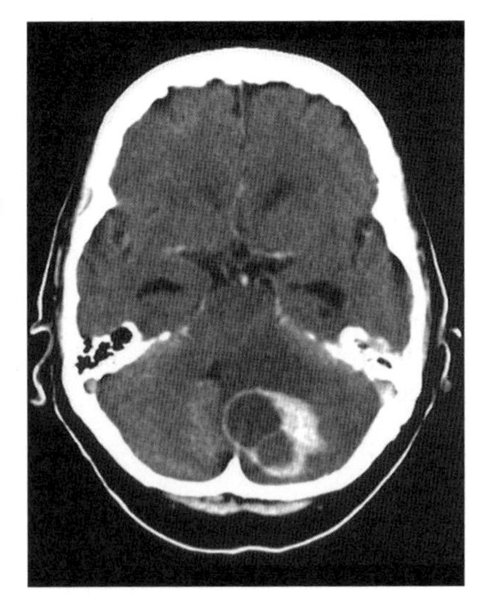

Haemangioblastomas (see Figure 23)

- Posterior fossa.
- Regular, well-circumscribed cystic.
- Hypodense but with isodense mural nodule.
- Mural nodule may enhance and become more clear.

Medulloblastomas

- Children.
- Posterior fossa, midline.
- Regular, well-circumscribed.
- Isodense.
- Homogeneous.
- Enhance homogeneously.

Ependymomas

- Mostly in children in the posterior fossa; also in adults and can appear anywhere in the brain.
- In the posterior fossa they usually arise from the foramina of Luschka and Magendie.
- Usually enhance uniformly.

Cerebellar gliomas

- Usually in children, and form the main differential diagnosis of posterior fossa tumours along with ependymomas and medulloblastomas.
- The same imaging characteristics are true as in the cerebral gliomas and they are usually not midline tumours.

Primitive neuroectodermal tumours (PNET)

- Found in the cerebrum in children.
- Have the same characteristics as medulloblastomas.

Dysembrioplastic neuroectodermal tumours

- Found in children and characterized by a very hypodense lesion almost the same density as CSF. No enhancement with contrast.

INFECTION (CEREBRITIS AND ABSCESS) (See Figure 24)

- Encapsulated abscess takes 2 weeks to develop from cerebritis.
- Cerebritis: normal scan or poorly defined hypodense area (may enhance).
- Abscess: well-defined rounded hypo/isodense lesion which 'ring-enhances' with contrast, with the capsule tending to be thinner on the side of the ventricle, and the side of the convexity being thicker.

CORTICAL INJURY

Diffuse axonal injury

- In acute stages, CT may be normal.
- Hyperdense spots (pettechial haemorrhages) in white matter – see the description of the three grades in the pathology section.

Cortical contusions

- Patchy areas of hypodensity with sporadic hyperdense spots (pettechial haemorrhages) in acute phase.
- Later, more hyperdense areas develop as bleeding continues and there is more associated hypodense oedema and mass effect; these lesions develop into haemorrhagic contusions, particularly between days 5 and 7, with maximal swelling and rebleeding occurring then.
- Temporal lobe and frontal lobes most commonly affected.

INFARCTION

- Normal scan in acute phase.
- Later, areas of low density develop and shape will depend on cause of infarction, e.g., wedge-shaped infarct with MCA occlusion but more diffuse areas with infarction after vasospasm associated with SAH.

SOME COMMON CYSTS

Arachnoid cyst

- Well-defined, hypodense extra-axial lesions (same density as CSF).
- Frequently found in the area of the pituitary fossa and cerebellopontine angle, but can be found anywhere.

Colloid cyst (see Figure 25)

- Small, round, hyperdense midline lesion in the anterior part of the 3rd ventricle.

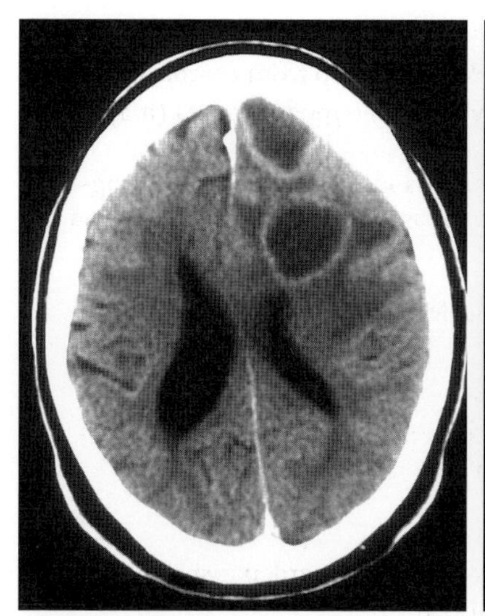

Figure 24. Axial CT scan with contrast, of two cerebral abscesses located in the left frontal lobe. The lesions are hypodense and ring-enhance with contrast.

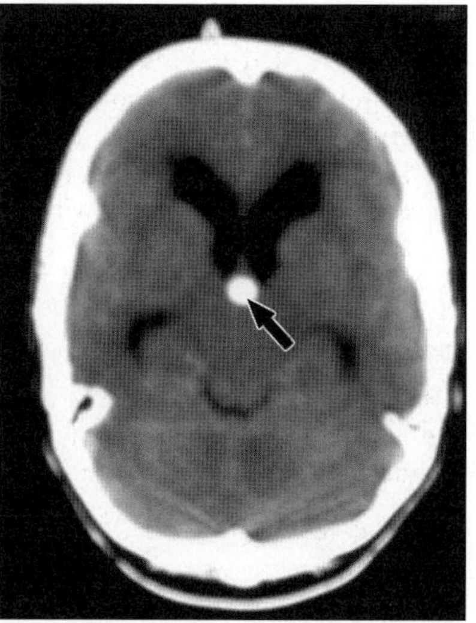

Figure 25. Axial CT scan showing a hyperdense colloid cyst in the anterior 3rd ventricle obstructing the foramen of Munro (arrow). Obstructive hydrocephalus is confirmed by the presence of distended anterior and temporal horns.

6

Overview of Neurosurgical Investigation and Monitoring

CONTENTS

INTRODUCTION

There are various specialist investigations relevant to neurosurgery and of which it will be helpful for SHOs to have a basic understanding. A brief overview follows of some of the more important specialist investigations you will come across.

MAGNETIC RESONANCE IMAGING

This is one of the new and exciting advances in neurosurgery and general imaging. The detailed physics behind this is quite complicated but essentially it is to align the spin of the molecules in tissue by a magnetic field and then to switch the field off and allow the molecules to return to their resting state. Different tissues allow the return to resting state at different speeds. By changing pulses of magnetism directed at these molecules returning to their resting state, all kinds of different image types can be generated. There are two times noted at the bottom of the scan: the first is the time to relaxation (TR), and the second the time to echo (TE), and the type of MRI scan is determined by these. This becomes a complicated business but there is a shortcut where just looking at the colour of the CSF will allow you to read MRI scans comfortably for the sequences that are used frequently.

T1 SEQUENCES

These are sequences that show water (and therefore CSF) as black. They are very good for demonstrating contrast enhancement, and taking out a T1 image from the MRI packet should be followed by taking out the T1 sequence with contrast administration (gadolinium – a paramagnetic substance) and putting it up next to compare whether there is any contrast enhancement. T1 sequences are usually used to identify cranial pathology, and it is common to have axial, sagittal and coronal cuts. Hyperintense lesions before contrast administration can only be fat, blood (acute stage) or melanin. Bone is hypointense, as is calcification. Brain tumours usually return less intense signals and are therefore hypointense (compare with hypodensity of CT scans). They usually have variable enhancement, with contrast becoming more hyperintense (compare hyperdensity of CT scans). The difference in nomenclature between CT and MRI scans is due to the fact that CTs function by the penetration of X-rays through tissues and we therefore talk about density, whereas the MRI scan works on the principle of the intensity of the returned signal of molecules in flux, hence we refer to it as intensity.

T2 SEQUENCES

In T2 sequences the CSF is white and tumours are usually white as well, reflecting the presence of fluid from cystic and necrotic areas as well as from neovascularization. These sequences are particularly useful when looking at spinal pathology since the white CSF makes a good contrast and backdrop to any pathology. Tumours or disc herniations can usually be seen to displace the normal white areas. Cranially, T2 sequences tend to overestimate the size of tumours, as the lesion seen is the tumour plus the surrounding oedema. A variation is the FLAIR sequence (fluid attenuated inverse ratio), which demonstrates only abnormal body water and not the normal anatomical CSF collections.

MAGNETIC RESONANCE ANGIOGRAPHY

Magnetic resonance angiography (MRA) is an excellent non-invasive tool, as is CT angiography (CTA). Both these modalities are noninvasive and are approaching the sensitivity and specificity of the gold standard, conventional digital subtraction angiography.

ANGIOGRAPHY

Conventional digital subtraction angiography is the gold standard for the detection of vascular abnormalities. New advances have been the ability to treat these abnormalities endovascularly and, potentially, to treat complications of SAH, such as vasospasm. There is a small but definite risk attached to this procedure; therefore it is not used as a routine screening test but only in cases where there is good reason to suspect underlying vascular abnormalities. You should know the basic anatomy on an angiogram and what

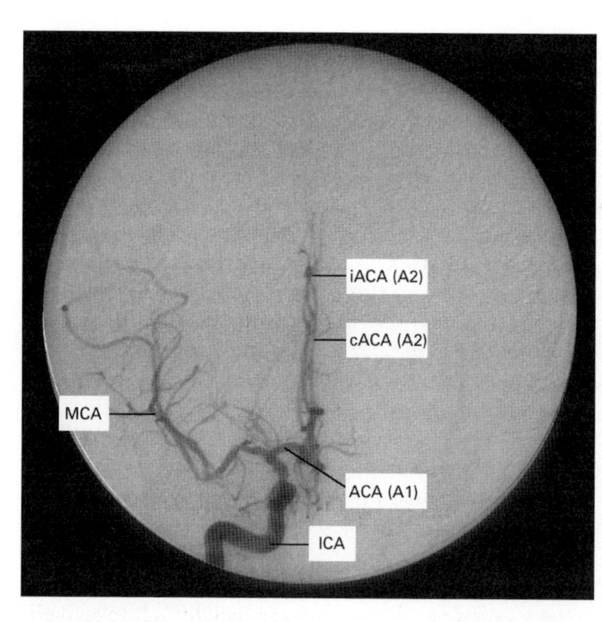

Figure 26. Right internal carotid angiogram sequence (postero–anterior view). The vessels are annotated as follows: middle cerebral artery, MCA; internal carotid artery, ICA; anterior cerebral artery A1 segment, ACA (A1); ipsilateral anterior cerebral artery A2 segment, iACA (A2); and contralateral anterior cerebral artery A2 segment, cACA (A2).

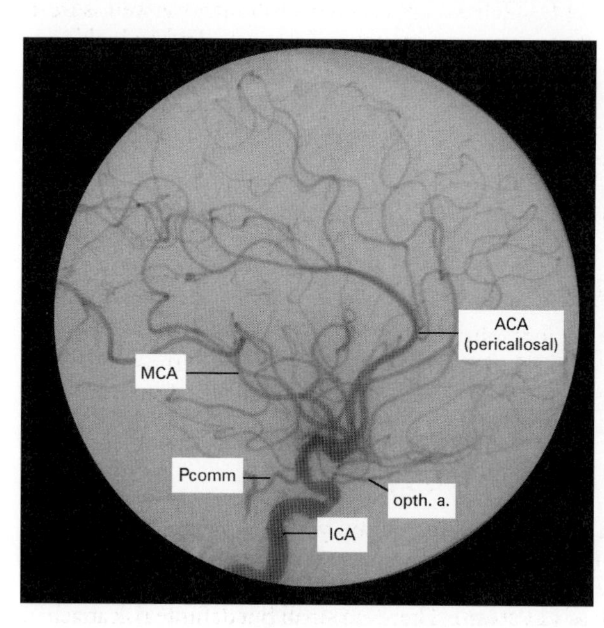

Figure 27. Right internal carotid angiogram sequence (lateral view). The vessels are annotated as follows: internal carotid artery, ICA; ophthalmic artery, ophth. a.; posterior communicating artery, Pcomm.; middle cerebral artery, MCA; anterior cerebral artery, ACA.

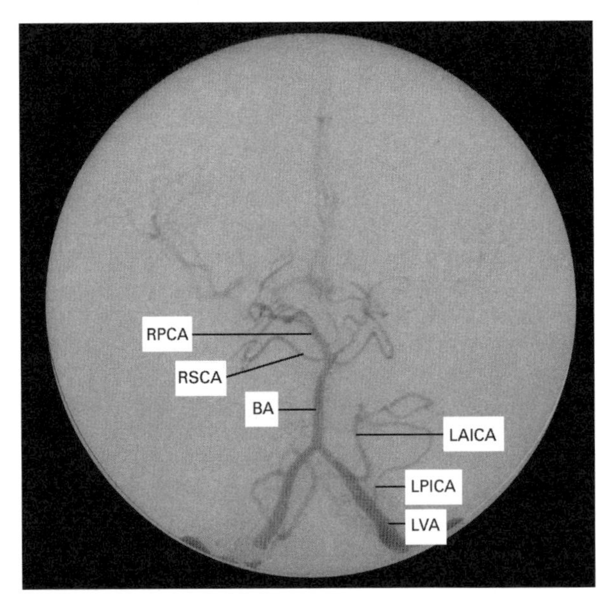

Figure 28.
Left vertebral artery angiogram sequence (anterior view). The vessels are annotated as follows: left vertebral artery, LVA; left posterior inferior cerebellar artery, LPICA; left anterior inferior cerebellar artery, LAICA; basilar artery, BA; right superior cerebellar artery, RSCA; right posterior cerebral artery, RPCA. Note that all these are paired, bilateral vessels, apart from the single midline basilar artery.

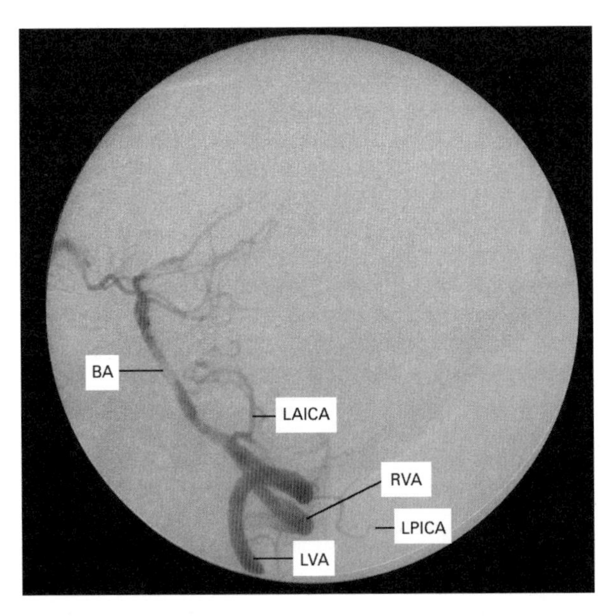

Figure 29.
Left vertebral artery angiogram sequence (lateral view). The vessels are annotated as follows: left vertebral artery, LVA; right vertebral artery, RVA; basilar artery, BA; left posterior inferior cerebellar artery, LPICA; left anterior inferior cerebellar artery, LAICA.

to look out for to be able to diagnose an AVM or aneurysm. There are usually several views done and they are marked in the top corner usually as LICA (left internal carotid artery), RICA (right internal carotid artery) and posterior circulation. There are AP and lateral views for LICA, RICA, and posterior circulation. See Figures 26, 27, 28 and 29 for examples of standard angiogram views.

Make sure that you can read the patient's name and that you have the two LICAs and two RICAs as well as the two posterior circulation sets together. There will also be an oblique or spin view of the LICA and RICA: ignore them for now.

What you need to do now is practise looking at the different arteries in the different views.

The internal carotid passes through the petrous bone and has several twists and turns before passing through the cavernous sinus and exiting through the foramen lacerum into the cranial space. It then has an ophthalmic segment, communicating segment, and a choroidal segment, before it divides into the middle cerebral artery (MCA) and anterior cerebral artery (ACA). The names of these segments are directly derived from the branches that leave the carotid.

The ophthalmic artery runs in an anterior direction and is the first branch seen. This is followed by the posterior communicating artery (Pcomm) slightly higher up, which joins up with the posterior cerebral artery. The Pcomm is usually slightly larger than the ophthalmic artery, but sometimes it is much larger and this is then called a fetal Pcomm. In the fetus, the posterior circulation is fed by the anterior circulation *via* the Pcomm and only later in fetal development is the posterior circulation fed by the vertebral arteries and the basilar artery. If this state persists, the Pcomm is hypertrophied and important in the supply of the posterior cerebral territory (occipital lobes).

The next artery is the anterior choroidal artery which is usually within 4 mm of the bifurcation of the carotid and also extends posteriorly. Aneurysms are flow-related phenomena and therefore are usually seen at the origin of these arteries rather than distally. Therefore, if you carefully follow the carotid up to the bifurcation, looking at the origins of the opthalmic, posterior communicating artery and the anterior choroidal arteries, you will not miss aneurysms (looking like round or irregular outpouchings) on these arteries. Do this for both the left and right sides.

On the lateral views there are two areas to look at now. One is the very busy area where the branches of the MCA are coming directly at us and are quite bundled together on the image, and the other is the area of the ACA, which curves anteriorly and around the corpus callosum and allows easy identification of the branches as they are seen on their lateral aspect. The ACA has a precommunicating segment, a communicating segment and a postcommunicating segment. The precommunicating segment is short and extends from the origin of the ACA to the anterior communicating artery (Acomm) which connects the two ACAs. Most aneurysms are found around the Acomm as this is where the most turbulent flow occurs as the arteries change direction. Distal to the communicating segment there are several branches: the frontopolar, callosomarginal, and pericallosal arteries. It is unusual for aneurysms to occur in these branches.

On the AP view, the MCA artery can be visualized properly and it has two bifurcations where aneurysms usually form: one proximal and the other more distal. This view will also demonstrate which ACA is the dominant artery and whether it flows across to the other ACA *via* the Acomm. This is important, since we usually approach an Acomm aneurysm from the nondominant hemisphere.

The posterior circulation should be filled by both vertebral arteries during angiography and an AP and lateral view is used to demonstrate aneurysms. Identifying AVMs can take some experience. Angiography is a dynamic process and there will be several images of the same view on one film. This is to demonstrate the filling of the arteries; the last images are the venous phase and start to show up the veins into which the arteries drain. Seeing a vein earlier than expected would mean a shortcut between the arterial and venous system and therefore an AVM. A blush of arteries and veins together can be quite easily seen, and this also denotes an AVM. It is sometimes necessary to demonstrate not only the two internal carotid arteries (ICAs) and two vertebral arteries (four-vessel cerebral angiography) but also the two-external carotid arteries (six-vessel cerebral angiography) when there is a suspicion that the arteries supplying the dura contribute to an AVM.

ICP MONITORING

There are three ways in which to monitor ICP: subdural, intraparenchymal, and intraventricular. Subdural bolts are the most frequently used and they are the least sensitive – but they carry the least risk of infection. Placing the sensor into the parenchyma increases the sensitivity and accuracy of the measurement but increases the risk of infection. Intraventricular monitoring *via* an EVD is the most reliable and allows the option of draining CSF off when there is an increase in ICP. The sensors are attached to a monitor and the pressures are recorded continuously. Normal CSF pressures differ from person to person but a pressure of more than 10 cm H_2O is abnormal and a pressure of more than 20 cm H_2O usually warrants treatment. Looking at the pressure waves on the monitor also gives us a lot of information. In cases where there are short, transient increases of ICP, the clinical effect is usually not severe. If there is a continuous increase or a plateau in ICP, it becomes important to treat it, as these are usually malignant increases. See the section on basic procedures for the insertion of an ICP bolt.

DUPLEX DOPPLER

This is a velocity measurement of blood flow, and is used to provide evidence of vasospasm. The MCA is usually targeted through the thin squamous temporal bone, but the Doppler technician can also target other intracranial arteries. If the blood flow exceeds 200 ml/s in the MCA, it is indicative of vasospasm. In the awake patient, clinical deterioration is usually the hallmark of vasospasm but duplex Doppler can diagnose vasospasm in the awake and comatose/sedated patient. It is therefore a valuable tool in the treatment of SAH patients.

JUGULAR VENOUS OXYGEN MONITORING

Continuously monitoring the amount of oxygen in the venous blood as it returns from the brain can help to tell us what the oxygenation of the brain parenchyma is like, and this procedure is used in some centres. The aim is to stop the oxygenation from dropping below 60% by manipulating the blood pressure and ventilation requirements. Few units use it routinely.

PERFUSION CT SCANNING

Perfusion CT scans are ordinary CT scans where contrast is administered and a software package calculates the perfusion in the different areas of the brain according to the flow of contrast through it. Other perfusion scans use the administration of xenon gas to calculate blood flow; these can demonstrate regional hypoperfusion states and allow us to modify our therapy.

POSITRON EMISSION TOMOGRAPHY

Only a very few centres have positron emission tomography (PET) as it requires a cyclotron. PET scans are functional scans which can detect radioactive isotopes which are administered to patients. Oxygen uptake and glucose delivery can demonstrate biological activity and, for instance, differentiate between a tumour or post-radiation necrosis, a distinction which is notoriously difficult to make by other means.

7
Ward Management of Neurosurgical Patients

CONTENTS

INTRODUCTION

Individual Consultants and different neurosurgical units will undoubtedly have their own preferences as to how to manage patients on the ward. However, it is unlikely that the management will differ drastically from that described below. This chapter is designed to give you an overview, and insight into what you are trying to achieve whilst managing patients on the ward. It cannot be overemphasized how important your input is on the wards. The whole unit is built around the nursing staff and the SHOs. The calibre of the current batch of SHOs is evidenced by how well the unit functions. You should take pride in owning the unit and consider the Registrars and Consultants as mere infrequent visitors. It should never be possible for them to know more about your patients than you do. Good perioperative care really does equate with good outcome.

PATIENT TRANSFER

It is important to be aware of the patients that are being transferred into the unit each day, as much can be done to pre-empt problems and facilitate care before patients actually arrive in the unit. Most units will have a list of patients due to come in from other hospitals. Make sure that, at the beginning of each day, you find out from the on-call Registrar which patients are due to come in and what the plan of action for each is. For some patients the plan may be to see and assess, whereas for others it may be that theatre is a near certainty unless the patient's condition is radically different from that described by the referring team.

It is recommended that you contact the SHO or Houseman looking after each patient in the referring hospital and check up on the patient's situation. A patient might have been on the list for some days and things could have changed considerably. It is useful to ascertain an update on the patient's clinical state and find out what treatment has been initiated. Has the patient with the SAH been started on adequate IV fluids? Has the patient with the brain tumour been started on steroids? Has aspirin been stopped on the patient with the posterior fossa tumour due for theatre tomorrow? Has the INR been checked on the patient with the subdural haematoma? Has the sodium been checked recently on the SAH patient?

For a patient being transferred as an emergency, it might be possible to arrange for cross-matched blood to be sent with the patient. For all patients, it is imperative that hard copies of their scans are sent with them. It is usually not possible to print films from an image link, and hard copies of films will be needed in theatre. This is extremely important as this will prevent delays in going to theatre and, in neurosurgery, time is life.

The following is a good check-list for a sure and safe transfer:

S Scans: have hard copies been sent with the patient?
U Update: has the patient's condition changed?
R Rx: what treatment has the patient received so far?
E Electrolytes: are all blood results available?

&

S Steroids: have steroids have been given (dose and duration)?
A Aspirin: if necessary, has aspirin been stopped?
F Fluids: has appropriate fluid regime been commenced?
E Extra investigations: CXR? Coag screen? PSA/ESR?

GENERAL PERIOPERATIVE CARE

CEREBRAL TUMOURS

Patients with cerebral tumours tend to present with a progressive history of headache, focal neurological deficit, or fits. Patients with signs of raised intracranial pressure or focal neurology will usually benefit from a course of steroids. A loading dose, e.g., 10 mg dexamathasone IV, can be given, followed by 4 mg dexamethasone (oral or IV) qds. This can be gradually reduced after surgery in most instances. If a patient deteriorates whilst on steroids due to further mass effect of the tumour then it is often worth trying another loading dose of 8–10 mg dexamethasone IV.

It is important to be overcautious with steroids, and to check with the Registrar what the exact plan is. Some patients may have their steroids reduced and stopped while others may be left on a maintenance dose of 2 mg dexamethasone bd orally, at least until seen by the oncologist. Patients cannot be left on steroids indefinitely, and as a general rule, patients are not usually discharged on steroids unless there is an express instruction from a senior to do so. Steroids have serious side effects including psychosis, and intracranial or intraspinal sepsis. All patients on steroids need to receive some form of protection against gastric ulceration, e.g., ranitidine or lansoprazole.

In patients with tumours without a tissue diagnosis it is essential to ensure that basic investigations have been performed to rule out a primary lesion outside the CNS. This means that a full history needs to be taken. A full clinical examination needs to be performed, including a breast examination in women. A chest X-ray to look for an obvious lung primary is a minimum requirement. Basic blood work should include a U&E, FBC, LFT, ESR and clotting studies in the form of an INR. If there is a suspicion of prostate carcinoma then a PSA can add useful extra information.

Check-list for cerebral tumours

1. Full Hx and Ex for primary tumour.
2. Steroids – loading dose (10 mg dexamethasone) and maintenance (4 mg dexamethasone qds).
3. CXR.
4. FBC, UE, INR (± PSA).
5. Operative plan – biopsy/debulk.
6. CT scans done and available on ward.

SUBARACHNOID HAEMORRHAGE

The ward management of SAH is a fine balance and also extremely important. A good operation is not the only surgical factor that determines a good outcome in SAH. A large part is due to your diligence and meticulous care on the ward. In an ideal world, all SAH patients would be best managed in a high-dependency environment. However, resources being what they are, many patients of good WFNS (World Federation of Neurosurgeons Scale) grade (see Chapter 13, Table 4) will, of necessity, be admitted to the neurosurgical ward prior to angiography and surgical treatment. It is important to have a clear idea of the risks these patients face and what you are trying to achieve perioperatively.

Patients face the greatest risk of a devastating rebleed in the first 24 h and the risk of rebleed is as high as 20% in the first 2 weeks following the initial event – with 4% rebleeding on the first day and 1.5% per day for the next 2 weeks. There is an 80% mortality with a rebleed. Blood often enters the ventricular system at the time of the initial bleed and patients may develop obstructive hydrocephalus due to blockage of CSF flow within the ventricular system (e.g., aqueduct or outlet of 4th ventricle) or communicating hydrocephalus due to blockage of reabsorption through the arachnoid granulations (this usually occurs at a later stage). If there is a large intraparenchymal blood clot, patients may deteriorate due to the mass effect. SAH patients are at high risk of developing vasospasm which is one of the major causes of neurological deficit and morbidity in this group (see Chapter 13, Table 5). The greatest risk of vasospasm after the initial bleed occurs around 1 week, especially days 4–7; the risk is low in the first 3 days and later than 2 weeks. Electrolyte abnormalities are common in SAH patients – in particular, hyponatraemia due to cerebral salt-wasting. There is a small but not insignificant risk of developing seizures following SAH. In summary, therefore, you need to be aware that patients admitted with SAH are specifically at risk of: (1) rebleeding; (2) hydrocephalus (usually obstructive in acute phase); (3) vasospasm (delayed); (4) hyponatraemia; (5) seizures. Your perioperative care is aimed at preventing these complications by reducing the risk of their happening.

Measures that need to be taken to prevent rebleeding include preventing excessive rises in blood pressure. This has to be balanced with preventing an excessive drop in blood pressure which might exacerbate vasospasm. The patient should be nursed in as quiet and calm an environment as possible and usually on strict bed rest. Be careful not to put patients in a corner of the ward that is quiet because it is not readily visible – when these patients do deteriorate you will need to act quickly. Patients may be better with 30° head up as, at least in theory, this may help in maintaining CSF flow, reduce ICP due to increased venous return and prevent chest problems in the more elderly patients. Remember that placing patients on bed rest increases their risk of developing deep-vein thromboses (DVTs), so TEDs should be prescribed. Medication is important in preventing large increases in blood pressure.

Adequate analgesia should be prescribed, e.g., a codeine phosphate infusion which can be titrated to the clinical response and helps to guard against a precipitous drop in blood pressure associated with some forms of intramuscular analgesia regimes. Antiemetics, and laxatives such as lactulose, help prevent the blood pressure changes associated with nausea and constipation, and should be prescribed. Oral nimodipine has been shown in randomized controlled trials to reduce delayed ischaemic deficits associated with vasospasm. The regime that should be used is 60 mg of nimodipine orally every 4 h, and this should be continued for 21 days after the initial bleed. If patients are unable to take oral medication then an IV infusion can be used instead.

SAH patients should be well hydrated with oral or IV fluids as this is thought to reduce the risk of vasospasm. At least 3 litres of fluid per day should be given; if this is done intravenously, then saline is preferable. Hydration is one of the 3 Hs of 'triple-H' therapy for vasospasm (see ICU section, Chapter 8, for further discussion). Daily electrolytes should be monitored with a close eye on the sodium to identify hyponatraemia early.

Routine blood work should include coagulation studies in the form of an INR and group and save (cross-match at least 4 units if the patient is going to have an aneurysm clipped).

Check-list for subarachnoid haemorrhage

1. Strict bed rest.
2. Nimodipine 60 mg 4-hourly.
3. 3 L fluids/day.
4. Analgesia – e.g., codeine phosphate infusion.
5. Lactulose 10 ml bd.
6. U&E, FBC, INR, X-match (daily Na+).
7. Hourly neuro-obs minimum.
8. CT scans available on ward.
9. Results of lumbar puncture (if done) written in notes.

HEAD INJURIES

You will see many patients with head injuries during your time as a neurosurgical houseman. In general, if a patient needs admission to a neurosurgical unit then the head injury is severe. Some patients will arrive and go directly to theatre for evacuation of a traumatic bleed (extradural or acute subdural haematomas) or exploration of depressed skull fractures. Others may be unconscious due to diffuse axonal injury or cerebral contusions and will be admitted to the ICU for ICP monitoring and care. There will also be a subgroup of patients with contusions or small intracranial haematomas who are considered at high risk of further deterioration and are, therefore, admitted to the neurosurgical unit for ICP monitoring and observation. If the condition of these patients deteriorates they will need rescanning and either theatre or ICU care.

The principles of head injury care are the same for all patients, and whilst all should have been assessed according to the ATLS protocol in the referring hospital, it is nevertheless essential that, on a patient's arrival in the neurosurgical unit, you reassess each patient according to the ATLS protocol, as the patient's situation may have changed.

If a patient is intubated and ventilated, check pupillary response. If bilaterally fixed dilated pupils are found, it may not be appropriate to undertake surgery. If the patient arrives unventilated then your assessment might determine the need for intubation. Remember: GCS less than 8 = intubate! If you are not happy with the safety of the airway, speak to your Registrar or the anaesthetist and ask about HDU/ICU care.

Ensure that, if the neck is not immobilized, the patient has had adequate C-spine clearance in the referring hospital. Find the C-spine films and determine whether they are adequate or not. If the patient is not sufficiently awake for clinical assessment of the C-spine do not be afraid to put a collar on the C-spine even if the neck films are normal. The patient's neck can be reassessed when they are more alert, or by further imaging. Ensure that you are happy with your primary survey before moving on to the secondary survey. If a full trauma series has not been undertaken then ensure that this is done. Check the notes for blood results – bloods may have been taken but perhaps not checked before transfers. Ensure that you have a sample of blood for cross-match.

Document your neurological assessment clearly to include GCS and pupil reactions. If a patient has deteriorated neurologically at any time then reassess everything again and discuss with the Registrar before sending the patient for another scan. Ask for a minimum of hourly neuro-obs from the nursing staff. Examine the scalp for wounds and see what management and care they have received. All wounds need to be cleaned properly. If there is an underlying depressed skull fracture, proper surgical exploration and debridement will be required in theatre. Check specifically for CSF leak from the nose and ears and document it.

There are several controversial issues in the management of head injuries. Are anticonvulsants indicated to prevent epilepsy? Should prophylactic antibiotics be given in the presence of CSF leak? Are steroids of any benefit in head injury? All these issues are discussed in the chapter on controversies and evidence base in neurosurgery. It is generally accepted that prophylactic antibiotics should not be given. If a patient is septic, however, then antibiotics are indicated after appropriate samples have been sent for culture. Discuss with your Registrar regarding choice of antibiotic, and never perform an LP without clearing it with a senior first. If there is an open skull fracture then it is arguable that antibiotics should be given to prevent osteomyelitis. Steroids are sometimes given, although there is scant evidence for the value of doing so. See the section on controversies in neurosurgery (Chapter 12), and read about the ongoing CRASH (Corticosteroid Randomization After Significant Head Injury) trial. The situation is no more clear-cut for anticonvulsants, but many people will give anticonvulsants prophylactically in the form of phenytoin – this is also discussed in the section on controversies in neurosurgery.

Check-list for head injury

1. On arrival in unit, reassess according to ATLS guidelines.
2. If the patient's condition has changed determine whether they need to be in a HDU/ICU.
3. If the patient is stable, ensure secondary survey complete, including all appropriate radiology (C-spine cleared? – up to 30% of severe head injuries have associated spinal injuries), and ensure all blood work has been done.
4. Document neurology and ensure regular neuro-obs performed.
5. Antibiotics not normally given prophylactically but if there is CSF leak or open skull fracture discuss with Registrar or Consultant.
6. Phenytoin may be given prophylactically, but again discuss preferences with Registrar or Consultant.
7. Steroids probably not indicated.
8. Bloods, including group and save, done.

SHUNT PATIENTS

CSF shunts problems are a common cause for admission to the neurosurgical unit. The commonest problems will be under-shunting of CSF (e.g., due to disconnection or blockage) and infection, although some patients will present with low-pressure headaches due to over-shunting. Patients present in a variety of ways, e.g.: headaches; deterioration in conscious level; confusion; focal neurological deficit; sepsis; or fits. Assessment of patients with a shunt problem requires detailed inquiry regarding the history of the shunt itself. What was the indication for the shunt? When and where was it put in? Has it ever needed to be revised, and, if so, which end was revised? Does this episode feel like any previous episodes of shunt problems? Patients usually know if they have a shunt problem and, when the patient is a child, always believe the parents – they are almost always right. Enquire about symptoms of raised intracranial pressure (headache, nausea and vomiting, fatigue, ataxia), sources of sepsis (urinary tract infections, respiratory tract infections), and any seizures.

When examining the patient be sure to inspect and palpate the shunt along its entire length, looking particularly for obvious gaps in the shunt and areas of inflammation. Examine for signs of raised intracranial pressure (papilloedema, VIth nerve palsy, upward gaze palsy, bulging fonatenelles in infants). Pumping and tapping of shunts is best left to the Registrar until you have been taught how to do these. A CT scan needs to be performed and, if possible, old scans should be obtained for comparison. A shunt series of plain films, should be requested, as this provides information about the location of the distal catheter and may identify any obvious disconnections. Blood work should include white cell count and inflammatory markers to look for evidence of an infective process.

Check-list for shunts

1. Full Hx & Ex.
2. CT scan + old films if available.
3. Shunt series.
4. WCC, ESR, CRP.
5. Shunt tap (never do this without discussing with Registrar/Consultant)

PITUITARY PATIENTS

To understand the perioperative care of patients with pituitary tumours it is helpful to consider briefly the effects these tumours may have. The mass effect of pituitary tumours can cause compression of: the optic chiasm, causing visual field defects; the pituitary gland, causing hypopituitarism; and the cavernous sinus, causing compression of cranial nerves III, IV, V_1, V_2, and VI. Pituitary tumours may be functional, secreting a variety of hormones, e.g., prolactin, adrenocorticotrophic hormone (ACTH), growth hormone (GH). It is essential, therefore, to examine and document visual fields and cranial nerves thoroughly. Formal visual field testing by an ophthalmologist is often organized preoperatively and should always be booked postoperatively. Blood work must include endocrine evaluation. Most Consultants will insist that the results of these endocrine investigations are documented in the notes. It is useful to discuss the appropriate blood tests with an endocrinologist early on in your job. Most Consultants will work in liaison with a particular endocrinologist, and getting to know them will greatly facilitate the care of your patients. In general, all pituitary patients will need preoperative assessments of prolactin and growth hormone levels, IgF1, testosterone, FSH, LH, and other profiles, to assess their adrenal, gonadal, and thyroid axes. Inducing the pituitary to produce cortisol with the short synacten test will indicate any occult deficiencies in the pituitary secretion of cortisol which might therefore be inadequate during a stress response. These patients need a low maintenance dose of cortisol. There is obviously also a high risk of disrupting pituitary function at surgery, and all patients will need steroid cover postoperatively. An example regime is 100 mg hydrocortisone IV at induction of anaesthesia, followed by 50 mg IV 8–12-hourly postoperatively, reduced gradually to 20 mg mane and 10 mg nocte, both orally, before discharge. Remember to give gastric cover with ranitidine or lansoprazole. Watch carefully for the development of diabetes insipidus (DI) by monitoring urine output and daily sodium levels (see below for management of DI). All pituitary patients need a follow-up endocrinology appointment and this should be booked and documented in the notes. Prophylactic antibiotics (amoxicillin and flucloxacillin) are commonly given in pituitary surgery as there will be contact of CSF with the nasal cavity. If a CSF leak is detected postoperatively, observe the patient carefully for the development of meningitis.

Check-list for pituitary patients

1. Formal visual field assessment and documentation of cranial nerve examination.
2. Pre-op endocrine assessment discussed with endocrinologist and results documented in notes.
3. Steroid cover from induction and reduced to maintenance post-op.
4. Antibiotic prophylaxis – watch for CSF leak and development of meningitis.
5. Monitor urine output and daily $Na+$ post-op.
6. Ophthalmology appointment booked.
7. Endocrinology follow up booked and documented in notes.

SPINAL PATIENTS

You will manage a range of spinal patients on the neurosurgical ward, including those with spinal injuries, acute compression syndromes, and patients admitted electively for laminectomies and discectomies. Patients with spinal injuries should be managed in a similar fashion to that described for head-injured patients, with a full reassessment on admission according to ATLS principles. If in doubt about C-spines, ensure that hard collars and sand bags are used. Spinal injury patients are at risk from aspiration and hypotension and so ensure that you are happy with the airway and pay close attention to the blood pressure (minimum IV line with saline infusion). Document the results of a detailed neurological examination, paying particular attention to motor and sensory levels. Document sacral sensation and sphincters (check anal tone and ask whether the patient can feel you pulling gently on their catheter). Steroids may have a role to play in spinal trauma (see later chapter on controversies and evidence in neurosurgery) and methylprednisolone should be given within 8 h of injury (30 mg/kg over 15 min with a 45 min pause, then 5.4 mg/kg/h for a least the first 24 h (48 h if started >3 h after injury). If a patient needs a fracture stabilized surgically, be sure to check with the operating surgeon regarding instructions for mobilization, e.g., to see whether any check films are required first.

Patients with spinal stenosis or disc prolapse may be admitted electively for surgery or as an emergency if there is rapidly progressive motor weakness, a cauda equina syndrome, or intractable pain. Again, it is important to document neurology, including the presence or absence of saddle anaesthesia and sphincter disturbances. Steroids, in the form of dexamethasone, are advocated in cases of spinal cord compression by some, but not all, neurosurgeons. In the postoperative period it is imperative to document any change in neurology and to check wounds regularly for CSF leak. In patients who undergo anterior approaches through the neck to cervical discs, keep an eye out for haematoma formation as there is a risk of airway compromise with haematomas in the neck. Spinal tumours should be managed in an analogous way to cerebral tumours and these patients will benefit from steroids (dexamethasone).

COMPLICATIONS

If at all possible, it is recommended that you try to attend a CCrISP course, as this provides you with a systematic approach to all surgical patients with complications on the ward. The principles are the same for neurosurgery but it is helpful if you are aware of and understand some of the complications which are specific to, or common in, neurosurgical patients.

'MRS JONES HAS DIPPED'

This is perhaps the commonest reason you will be called to the ward – because a patient has 'dipped'. Be sure to ascertain what is meant by 'dipped'. It usually refers to a drop in the GCS, or to a deterioration in focal neurology. Go and assess the patient and remember to use an ABCDE approach as neurosurgical patients need system support and can deteriorate from cardiorespiratory problems, such as myocardial infarctions (MIs), pulmonary embolisms (PEs) and chest infections, as much as any other surgical patient. While you are giving oxygen and putting in your lines, find out about the patient's diagnosis and treatment and try to have a list of reasons why a neurosurgical patient might 'dip' neurologically. The following is a useful check-list:

Post-op craniotomy

1. Haematoma –EDH, ASDH, intraparenchymal.
2. Cerebral oedema.
3. Fits.
4. Na+ abnormalities.
5. Infection – meningitis/abscess.
6. Hydrocephalus

Cerebral tumour patients

1. Further mass effect and oedema.
2. Fits.
3. Bleed associated with tumour.

SAH patients

1. Rebleed.
2. Hydrocephalus.
3. Vasospasm.
4. Na+ abnormalities.

Patients with shunts or EVDs

1. Shunt/EVD failure
2. Meningitis
3. Fits

Head injuries

1. Blossoming of contusions.
2. Further bleeding – EDH, ASDH.
3. Fits.
4. Meningitis.
5. Na^+ abnormalities.

Remember to consider rapidly reversible causes, such as low blood glucose and fits. Patients who have fitted may be postictal. Do not be afraid to use lorazepam to control patients who are actively fitting, but beware of using sedatives in patients who are postictal. If in doubt, there is little harm in loading patients with phenytoin (15–18 mg/kg loading dose over at least 30 min to prevent cardiac dysrythmias. Maintenance is 5–8 mg/kg/day in single night-time dose or divided doses over the day). Once you are happy that a patient is stable from a cardiorespiratory perspective (this may mean asking the anaesthetist to intubate) then the patient will need some form of repeat imaging, probably in the form of a CT scan. Always inform the Registrar on-call about patients who 'dip' as they may require theatre urgently. Figure 30 summarizes the sequence of actions in a patient whose level of consciousness drops on the ward.

CSF LEAKS

CSF leaks may occur after trauma or surgery. CSF leaks from surgical wounds may stop with an extra stitch or two. Patients with CSF leaks following spinal surgery can be placed on bed rest for a few days to reduce the effect of gravity and allow the wound to heal. It is essential to check operative notes and postoperative instructions as there may be a documented breach of the dura at the time of surgery. Antibiotics are not usually given prophylactically for CSF leaks. In patients who develop subcutaneous CSF collections following craniotomy, a lumbar drain is sometimes inserted. Beware being asked to undertake repeated aspirations of CSF collections. There is a significant risk of introducing infection and if there is no bone flap under the scalp you need to be careful not to damage the brain. There is no right or wrong answer in managing CSF collections, and Consultants will have their own methods based on their own experiences. If a patient with a CSF leak develops signs of sepsis discuss lumbar puncture and antibiotic treatment with your Registrar or Consultant.

DEEP-VEIN THROMBOSIS (DVT)

Remember that patients on bed rest are at risk of DVTs and require TEDs and possible anticoagulant prophylaxis. In the neurosurgical population, 30% of patients develop DVTs, although the majority will be asymptomatic.

Check with the Registrar or Consultant before starting anticoagulants, as you need to balance the risk of intradural haematoma with risk of DVT.

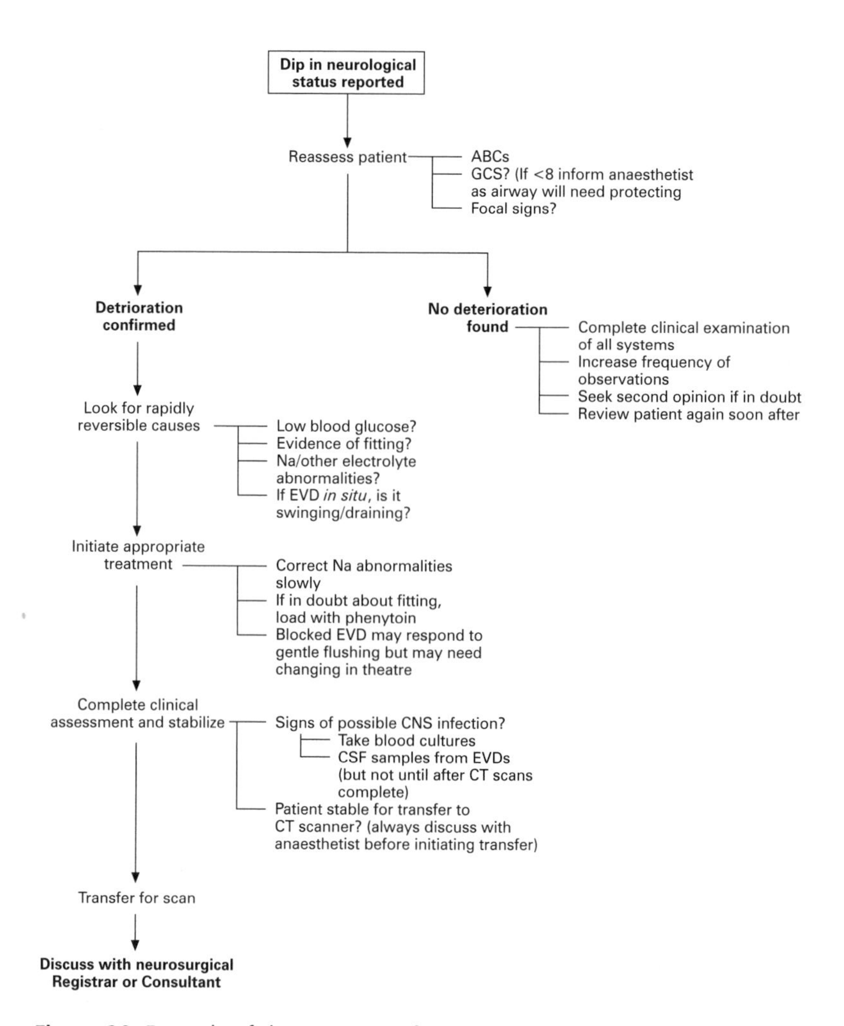

Figure 30. Example of the sequence of actions in a patient who 'dips' on the ward, i.e., a deterioration in neurological status is reported. Although there is no single correct sequence of events, this chart highlights various essential points, including the need to consider and, if necessary, treat reversible causes of neurological deterioration before sending a patient to the CT scanner.

Most Consultants will be comfortable with anticoagulants more than 48 h after surgery. There is literature demonstrating that using low-dose heparin preoperatively and directly postoperatively in craniotomy leads to no increased risk of haemorrhage.

SODIUM ABNORMALITIES

There are several conditions which are frequently seen in neurosurgical patients and which cause abnormalities in serum sodium. You need to be able to recognize them and be familiar with their treatment. Raised serum sodium is seen in diabetes insipidus (DI), and reduced sodium is seen in cerebral salt wasting (CSW) and the syndrome of inappropriate antidiuretic hormone secretion (SIADH). It is particularly important to understand the differences between CSW and SIADH because, although both produce hyponatraemia, they have different effects on extracellular fluid volumes and are treated differently. Remember that all abnormalities of sodium, particularly low sodium, need to be corrected slowly and cautiously due to the risk of central pontine myelinosis.

Diabetes insipidus

Reduced ADH secretion is known as neurogenic DI, whereas renal resistance to ADH is known as nephrogenic DI. Neurogenic DI is the type you are most likely to encounter in neurosurgical patients and may be the result of trauma, tumours, infection, or surgery. Patients at particular risk are those with severe head injury involving damage to the pituitary, after pituitary surgery, or with lesions pressing on the pituitary (e.g., craniopharyngiomas or anterior communicating artery aneurysms). It is important to appreciate that DI may be transient, especially after pituitary surgery. Because of the reduction in ADH there is production of a large volume of dilute urine (>200 ml/h, urine osmolality <200 mosm/kg). As a consequence the serum sodium rises (>145 mmol/l with plasma osmolarity >295 mosm/kg). In conscious patients this will result in a thirsty patient who classically craves iced water. The volume of fluids taken in may be enough to match losses and keep serum sodium within the normal range. This is where most cases of DI are missed. It is assumed that the high urine output is due to polydipsia. The key issue, therefore, is whether or not the kidneys are concentrating urine. A quick bedside test is to dip the urine to test specific gravity. Urine in DI will have a specific gravity <1.005; if it is >1.010, then the patient almost certainly does not have DI. In patients with suspected DI always check specific gravity, serum and urine sodiums and osmolalities. If DI is mild then patients may be able to keep up with fluid losses by taking fluid orally. If DI is more severe, or if the patient is not able to drink because of reduced conscious level, then IV fluids will need to be administered. In this situation dextrose is preferable to saline as the serum sodium is likely to be high. In transient DI, chasing fluid losses until the episode resolves is the best management. However, when it is proving difficult to keep up with losses the ADH analogue DDAVP may need to be given. This should be used cautiously and only with senior supervision. There is a danger that, if DDAVP is given inappropriately in too high doses, urine output can dry up, with resultant renal shut-down and no urine production, leading to brain swelling and a serious situation. Although the subcutaneous dose is 1–4 μg, we usually start at a lower dose of 0.5 μg or even less.

Cerebral salt wasting

Cerebral salt wasting (CSW) can be defined as renal loss of sodium secondary to intracranial disease. The physiological basis for renal sodium loss is unknown, but it is likely that there is an as yet unidentified natriuretic factor involved. CSW results in hyponatraemia and is also associated with loss of water. This is in contrast to SIADH (see below), in which there is hyponatraemia-associated retention of water due to excess ADH. CSW is seen particularly in patients with SAH. It is essential not to mistake CSW for SIADH in this setting, as fluid restriction (treatment for SIADH) in patients with SAH can precipitate or worsen vasospasm. To differentiate CSW from SIADH look at the patient's hydration (dry in CSW), CVP (low in CSW), and serum osmolality (normal or high in CSW, low in SIADH). CSW is treated by replacing fluid losses with salt-rich fluids: 0.9% or hypertonic saline. A very effective alternative or adjunctive is fludrocortisone, a mineralocorticoid which may need to be given to stimulate renal reabsorption of sodium; this should, however, be a senior decision.

Syndrome of inappropriate antidiuretic hormone secretion

SIADH can occur with a variety of neurosurgical pathology: tumours; head injury; post-craniotomy; meningitis. Inappropriate secretion of ADH results in hyponatraemia due to water retention. Serum sodium and serum osmolalities are, therefore, low but there is no detectable abnormality in renal function. Fluid restriction to <1 L/day is the first-line treatment. The use of hypertonic saline with diuretics should be reserved for refractory cases and undertaken only with senior advice. Remember the warning given above about confusing SIADH and CSW in patients with SAH.

FITS

Fits are a common complication in neurosurgical patients, and patients in status epilepticus need to be stopped from fitting. In status epilepticus, attention must be given to the airway and oxygen administered. Lorazepam 4 mg IV over 2 min can be given for adults actively fitting. If there is difficulty in obtaining IV access then PR benzodiazepines may be administered. Patients should be loaded with phenytoin 1 g IV even if the lorazepam/diazepam stops the fitting. If fitting still does not stop after phenytoin, call for senior assistance and consider phenobarbitone. Patients who require phenobarbitone to stop fitting generally need a short period on the HDU/ICU where they can be intubated and anaesthetized if necessary. If patients are anaesthetized to control their fits, it is important to obtain a continuous EEG tracing to determine whether or not seizure activity has been controlled – propofol might keep a patient quiet but it may not necessarily stop epileptic activity. Once seizure activity has been controlled, ensure that you initiate the relevant investigations. Check electrolytes and, if the patient was already on phenytoin, check the level. Consider rescanning the patient, as the intracranial picture may have changed, e.g., the devel-

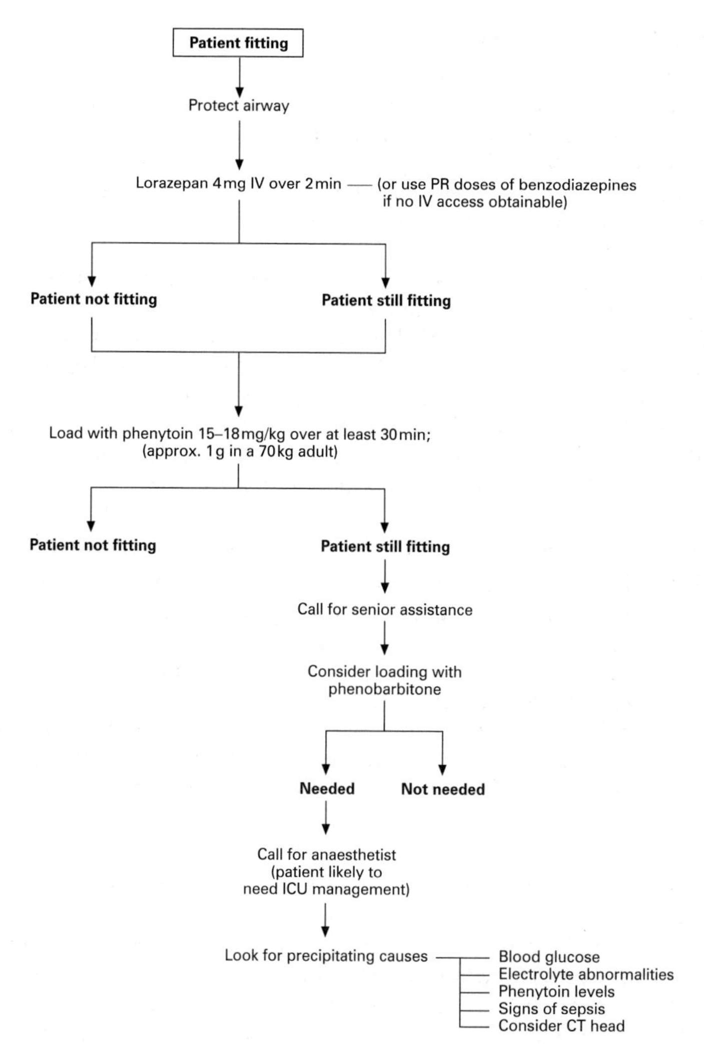

Figure 31. Management of the fitting patient (NB: doses will be different for paediatric patients).

opment of an EDH after a craniotomy. The basics of managing a fitting patient are summarized in Figure 31.

With an isolated fit consider loading the patient with phenytoin or discuss with a senior regarding alternatives. Again, initiate appropriate investigations and consider rescanning the patient.

8
ICU Management

CONTENTS

INTRODUCTION

The neuro-ICU can be a very daunting setting, particularly for someone who has not worked in an intensive-care unit before. The level of involvement of the SHO will depend upon both the neurosurgical unit and upon the SHO. In some units the role of the SHO will be limited to documenting the ward round in the notes. In other units the SHO may be more involved in the decision-making process and in the practical procedures on the unit. This chapter is designed to help those who are coming to neuro-ICU as a surgical SHO for the first time. The following outline of some of the key elements that are important to the neurosurgeon in the management of ICU patients will facilitate understanding of the issues discussed on the ICU rounds. This chapter is not a detailed discussion on how to be an ICU physician. Rather, it aims to serve as a guide in the first month or so of the job. The chapter has been divided into several sectionss that we feel will help you to understand what happens in a neuro-ICU.

DECISION-MAKING AND REVIEW ON THE NEURO-ICU

The first point to make is that, whatever your role in the decision-making process, you should always consider whether the right decision is being made for the patient. It may seem obvious, but it is imperative to remember that the whole aim of ICU management is to help the patient. The reason for making this seemingly obvious statement is that it is all too easy to get lost in correcting parameters. We would urge you to practise good patient care, not to perform physiological experiments. Remember the old adage – treat patients, not numbers.

The neuro-ICU consists of a team of surgeons, anaesthetists, and ICU-nursing staff. It is not possible to be an expert in everything and so it is imperative to coordinate and pool expertise needed for patient care. Anaesthetists are usually better than surgeons with applied respiratory physiology. Senior ICU-nursing staff are also extremely knowledgeable. Don't be afraid to ask any member of the team for advice. The ICU-staff will have much more experience than you and will be more than willing to share it with you.

In the neuro-ICU setting it is often thought that the only role of the neurosurgeon is to decide when, and when not, to operate, and to manage ICP. Although this is a very narrow and limited view, it does describe the area of neuro-ICU in which the neurosurgeons will be expected to know more than the rest of the team. However, it is good practice to be actively involved with the intensivists in the care of the whole patient. After all, there is no point deciding to operate on a patient who will not survive an anaesthetic because of their systemic illness. The following system of review for each patient on the ICU ward round will ensure that all problems are identified. For each patient you see on the ICU round consider the following six issues.

AIRWAYS AND NEUOLOGICAL STATUS

What is the patient's GCS? Is it good enough for the patient to maintain their own airway? If it is less than 8 then intubation will probably be necessary – inform and discuss with the anaesthetist. If the neurological status has changed then consider why it may have changed. What can be done to reverse the change? Will the patient need another scan? (but do not send the patient to the scanner until completely reviewed and deemed stable enough for transfer to the scanner). Does the patient need ICP monitoring? If there is an ICP monitor in already, is the ICP stable, and what, if anything, needs to be done? Are there any other airway issues? For example, if the patient has been intubated for a long period of time, do they need a tracheostomy? If a tracheostomy is in place, find out whether it is working and look for any complications. Is the patient sedated? If so, does the patient need to remain sedated or is it time to wean sedation (this will also depend on the condition of the patient's chest). Are there any spinal issues which have been overlooked?

BREATHING AND CHEST

Most ICU patients will be ventilated and are prone to developing chest infections. Patients who have been victims of trauma may have chest injuries requiring chest drains or that are undiagnosed. Find out from the anaesthetic team the condition of the chest and whether the patient would be fit to wean if neurologically stable. If the patient is not fit to wean from a chest point of view, find out whether anything can be done to improve respiratory function.

CIRCULATION

Is the patient cardiovascularly stable? Does the patient require inotropic support? If so, make sure that this is reviewed and the reasons for cardiovascular problems discussed. Review haematological investigations.

SYSTEMATIC REVIEW AND INVESTIGATIONS OF OTHER SYSTEMS

Review the patient's other systems: renal and hepatic physiology, for example. Check all blood results including glucose levels, electrolytes, haematology, and imaging.

SEPSIS

Many ICU patients will develop an infection of some kind. It is important, therefore, to spend a few minutes looking for evidence of infection in each patient. Ensure that the results of any culture specimens are chased up.

COMMUNICATION

Write a plan in the notes and include the bleep and name of the person who needs to be notified of the results of any investigation ordered. It is also essential to communicate with the family of neuro-ICU patients as they usually cannot do this themselves. Find out who spoke to the family last, and when. Make a plan to discuss any new changes with the appropriate relatives. For example, a typical plan might read as follows:

1. Continue current cardiorespiratory support.
2. CT head scan.
3. Inform neuro-Registrar on call (Bp 445) of CT result (patient may be for weaning).
4. Continue current antibiotics until cultures back.
5. Dr Wellgood to inform relatives of patient's status (unchanged)

MANAGEMENT OF ICP

Perhaps the main challenge to the neurosurgeon in the neuro-ICU is to prevent cell death of the different tissues making up the nervous system. Cells die due to tissue hypoxia, and tissue hypoxia is closely tied in with dyshomeostasis of the intracranial space. The brain has an excellent autoregulatory mechanism which keeps the blood flow to the tissues constant despite fluctuations in blood supply. This is true for cerebral perfusion pressures (CPP) between 50 and 150 mmHg. The main driving force for brain perfusion is the cerebral perfusion pressure and this is a combination of the positive effects of the mean arterial pressure (MAP) driving the blood forward and the negative effects of the ICP functioning as a resisting force. Therefore, if we can keep blood pressures within these limits, the brain tissues will be well perfused. We can calculate the CPP by subtracting the ICP in mmHg from the MAP in mmHg (CPP = MAP – ICP). The main aim is to keep the CPP at 70 mmHg, and this can be done by increasing the MAP as the ICP rises. For instance, an ICP of 20 necessitates a MAP of 90 mmHg. The brain usually undergoes damage if there is a sustained ICP of more than 20 mmHg. Therefore, the parameters that we usually use are: a CPP above 70 mmHg, a MAP of >90 mmHg and an ICP of <20 mmHg. Autoregulation is lost in many types of pathology, especially in severely injured patients. The protective measures of the brain are just completely overrun in these situations and no treatment seems to be able to bring the ICP down; as the brain loses its autoregulation mechanism, the perfusion of the brain becomes directly dependent on the MAP. Therefore, high blood flows will lead to hyperaemia and low blood flows to ischaemia. The MAP can be controlled in conjunction with the anaesthetist by ensuring, in cases of hypotension, that the patient has adequate intravascular volume according to CVP or wedge pressure measurement, and, if necessary, is placed on inotropes. In cases of hypertension – usually in excess of 200 mmHg – nimodipine, nitrates, β-blockers, diuretics and ACE-inhibitors can all be used. ICP is increased by the following factors, each of which will be considered in turn: hyperthermia; hypermetabolism; hyperglycaemia; increased venous pressure; hypercarbia; and increased plasma osmolality.

HYPERTHERMIA

Hyperthermia has a direct correlation with increased ICP and can be difficult to control at times. Normal antipyretics and external cooling with a cooling blanket to 35.5 °C is effective.

HYPERMETABOLISM

The ICP is increased by convulsions and in the actively moving restless patient, and therefore all patients should be actively sedated and seizures aggressively terminated.

HYPERGLYCAEMIA

The majority of neuro-ICU patients will need to be on a sliding scale to control their glucose level, since this contributes to the osmolality of the plasma and can lead to build up of lactic acid. At high levels of plasma glucose the glucose can cross the damaged blood–brain barrier and when water passively follows this gradient, brain oedema can result.

INCREASED VENOUS PRESSURE

High ventilation pressures and increased abdominal pressures lead to an increase in the venous outflow resistance and increased ICP.

HYPERCARBIA

Fluctuations in CO_2 concentration can have profound effects on ICP. Excess CO_2 causes vasodilatation and a low CO_2 leads to vasoconstriction. The Monroe-Kelly doctrine states that, if the blood flow increases, there has to be a compensatory decrease in the space occupied by the CSF and brain tissue. Since CSF dispersion is usually already a feature, the brain tissue undergoes compression. It has been found that hyperventilating patients is very effective in lowering the ICP *via* vasoconstriction. However, vasoconstriction leads to lower blood flow and the obvious complication of this is a possibility of ischaemia and infarction. A low normal pCO_2 of around 4.5–5 kPa is usually maintained to obtain the beneficial effects of vasoconstriction without impairing tissue perfusion. In adults, the positive effects of hyperventilation are negated after 24–48 h by compensatory renal mechanisms. Hyperventilation to produce CO_2 levels below 4.5 is reserved for the acute setting in patients who have rapidly decompensated and who are awaiting evacuation of a mass lesion.

PLASMA OSMOLALITY

Sodium is the main predictor of serum osmolality, and should be kept in the normal range at all times. Low sodium can be an indicator of fluid retention and intravascular overload which leads to increased vascular volumes and increased ICP. High sodium is an indicator of intravascular dehydration and leads to seizure activity, brain ischaemia and infarction. Sodium homeostasis is controlled by the hypothalamus and pituitary and so, not surprisingly, haemorrhage, infarctions, tumours or trauma in that area can lead to dyshomeostasis with fluid and sodium imbalance. See the chapter on the ward management of patients and particularly the section on the syndrome of inappropriate ADH secretion, cerebral salt wasting and diabetes insipidus.

A STEPWISE APPROACH TO DEALING WITH INCREASED ICP

A multitude of factors influence ICP, and we have to make sure that we follow a logical and stepwise approach to a patient on the ICU with increased ICP. Consider a patient who is comatose, intubated and ventilated on the neuro-ICU. They have an ICP monitor in place and the ICP goes up to 35. In this situation you need to get senior help from your Registrar, because one of the first steps will be to exclude a surgically reversible cause, e.g., intracranial haemorrhage, infarction or CSF build-up, by doing a CT scan as an emergency. However, it is essential to ensure that the patient is as stable as possible before transfer. If there is no surgically reversible cause seen on CT, medical management of the ICP will form the mainstay of treatment. The following points will need to be checked:

1. Is the patient adequately sedated with adequate pain relief and, if necessary, paralysed?
2. Are the ventilation pressures less than 20 mmHg and is the pCO_2 in the preferred range?
3. Is the patient normothermic to slightly hypothermic?
4. Seizures are usually clinically evident but in the paralysed patient can be subclinical. Their presence can be ascertained by doing an EEG. It is important to control seizures to prevent brain damage and raised ICP, irrespective of whether there are external manifestations of these seizures.
5. CSF drainage. If the patient has an EVD *in situ*, the safest and best way to reduce ICP is to drain off CSF. This is done by setting the drain at a pressure level that you do not want to be exceeded. If the drain is at 15 cmH_2O, CSF will drain off at any pressure higher than that. This is the usual level at which to set the pressure, but in different cases the drains will be put at different heights. For instance, in patients with communicating hydrocephalus following haemorrhage, the drain will be progressively raised to see whether a patient is drain-dependent or not.
6. Initiating a diuresis (Monroe–Kelly again). The osmotic diuretic, mannitol, is extremely effective in reducing ICP. It is even more effective when combined with a small dose of frusemide. The usual dose of mannitol would be 0.5–1 g/kg of body weight. This usually equates to about 100–200 ml of a 20% mannitol solution and the usual dose of frusemide to add would be 20 mg. Not only does mannitol cause an osmotic diuresis but it also improves the rheology of the blood, allowing easier brain perfusion, and it also acts as a free radical scavenger.

7. Initiating burst suppression on EEG scans, or even a flat line, the use of the barbiturate pentothal can slow down the metabolism of the brain. This is an effective therapy but is controversial since it causes the patient to be completely flat, with nonreacting pupils for a week or more after the pentothal is stopped. This is a last resort.
8. Decompressive craniectomies or craniotomies are also options to try in order to reduce the ICP. In patients in whom the ICP is refractory to all medical treatment, this can be life-saving. The bone is removed and stored for later replacement. This is the only treatment that counteracts the Monroe–Kelly principle by changing the anatomically limiting tissue from hard bone to more pliant soft tissue.

MANAGEMENT OF VASOSPASM

Vasospasm is a term in which is commonly used to denote the process by which the phenomenon of delayed ischaemic neurological deficit (DIND) is thought to be brought about. Although vasospasm is mostly associated with spontaneous SAH, it can occur in other situations, e.g., following other forms of intracranial bleeding, head injury, or intracranial surgery. However, as it will be primarily encountered in patients with SAH it will be discussed in this context. It is important to realize that vasospasm is one of the major causes of morbidity and mortality in SAH patients who survive long enough to be admitted to neurosurgical units. As discussed in the previous chapter, the greatest risk of vasospasm after the initial bleed is around 1 week, especially days 4–7, and vasospasm is rare in the first 3 days and later than 2 weeks. It is usually identified as a delayed deterioration in neurological status. This can either be a new focal neurological deficit (speech disturbances, motor deficits) or a reduction in the GCS. The situation is more complex in patients who are sedated and ventilated, as it will be almost impossible to identify any change in neurological status. In these patients angiography may reveal vasospasm. However, angiography has been found to identify vasospasm in patients without any neurological deficits and so its use and interpretation requires an experienced and cautious clinician.

Patients on the neuro-ICU can deteriorate for many reasons. It is essential, therefore, to rule out other causes of neurological deterioration before making a diagnosis of vasospasm. It will be necessary to consider other causes such as hydrocephalus, rebleed, seizures, electrolyte abnormalities, hypoglycaemia, and sepsis. If vasospasm is suspected, therefore, various investigations will need to be done (CT head scan, bloods for electrolytes, EEG if available, blood glucose levels). Ideally, for a diagnosis of vasospasm to be made, other causes of neurological deterioration should be excluded, the deficit should be present at the appropriate time (i.e., between 4 and 20 days after the initial bleed), and spasm should be confirmed by angiography (if available).

In addition to the overall supportive care provided by ICU, the mainstay of management for cerebral vasospasm is 'triple-H' therapy: hypervolaemia;

hypertension; and haemodilution. The use of fluids will help achieve all three Hs. However, pressors may be necessary to increase systolic blood pressure. Therapy is titrated to reverse neurological deficits, or in ventilated and sedated patients to reverse radiological spasm. Careful cardiovascular monitoring will be required for successful therapy. Also, it is important to be aware of the risks of triple-H therapy. In patients with an unprotected (unclipped or uncoiled) aneurysm there is an increased risk of rebleed. In patients with a large area of infarcted brain there is a risk of cerebral oedema.

Where triple-H therapy is unsuccessful, endovascular treatments may be used, e.g., angioplasty or intra-arterial papaverine. However, there are risks associated with endovascular methods, including arterial rupture and displacement of aneursym coils and clips.

HERNIATION SYNDROMES

If the ICP is not controlled then there will be herniation of brain tissue. It is useful, therefore, to be familiar with the different brain herniation syndromes.

TRANSTENTORIAL HERNIATION

There are four different transtentorial herniation syndromes:

Downward transtentorial herniation

The temporal lobes are squeezed downward through the tentorial incisura and this causes the medially protruding uncus to compress the brain stem and the surrounding structures. The ipsilateral third nerve is compressed and this leads to an ipsilateral dilated pupil. The ipsilateral cerebral peduncles are compressed, and because the motor fibres only cross lower in the medulla this leads to a contralateral hemiparesis.

Kernohan's paralysis

This involves an ipsilateral dilated pupil as well as an ipsilateral hemiparesis. This occurs when the ipsilateral uncus pushes the brainstem over and the contralateral cerebral peduncle is compressed against the tentorial hiatus, leading to compression of the contralateral cerebral peduncle and, following the decussation of the fibres, to an ipsilateral hemiparesis.

Upward transtentorial herniation

This occurs when a posterior fossa mass or bleed allows the cerebellum to herniate upwards through the tentorial incisura. The cerebellum causes fatal compression by posterior pressure on the brainstem.

Posterior cerebral artery compression

Another effect of transtentorial herniation is compression of the posterior cerebral artery as it courses next to the brainstem and curls over the edge of the tentoriun cerebelli and the tentorial incisura. This leads to infarction of the occipital cortex and cortical blindness with intact pupillary responses.

SUBFALCINE HERNIATION

Swelling of a hemisphere leads to herniation of that hemisphere underneath the rigid falx and resultant compression of the ventricular system. This leads to obstructive hydrocephalus and compression of the distal anterior cerebral artery branches, such as the pericallosal arteries, thereby causing infarcts in the territory supplied by those arteries.

CENTRAL HERNIATION

Herniation of the brain stem through the foramen magnum leads to compression of the medulla and the cardiorespiratory centres contained therein. This leads to arrhythmias (and possible cardiac arrest) and abnormal breathing patterns. Ataxic breathing is characterized by irregular depth and frequency of breathing in a random manner. Apneustic breathing is when there are long periods of no respiratory activity, and Cheyne–Stoke's breathing is characterized by increasing depth and frequency of breathing followed by an apnoeic period; this is repeated over and over. These are all preterminal signs, and at this stage patients are usually GCS 3/15 with nonreactive pupils. The cardiac warning signs are those of the Cushing response, with bradycardia and hypertension.

BRAIN DEATH AND BRAINSTEM TESTING

Patients are said to be brain dead when there is no brainstem function ascertainable. The following tests confirm brain death and should be performed by two doctors who have been registered for at least 5 years.

- The absence of any sedation or paralysing agents.
- Normothermia.
- Normal biochemistry.
- No motor response to central painful stimuli (press on the superior orbital rim in the mid-pupillary line to stimulate the supraorbital nerve).
- No pupillary light response.
- No corneal reflex.
- No doll's eye reflex. Test by holding the eyes open and, elevating the head 30°, rotate the head rapidly from left to right. People who are alive fix on a certain point but in people who are dead the eyes remain staring in their heads exactly the same as in a doll.
- Caloric testing is done by injecting ice-cold water into the ear and stimulating the eardrum whilst holding the eyes open. In people with functioning brainstems this leads to nystagmus.

- No gag reflex. Test by suctioning or pulling on the ET tube or externally stimulating the larynx.

Apnoea testing is the last and definitive test. This is done by pre-oxygenating a patient on 100% oxygen, then disconnecting the patient from the ventilator and passing a catheter down the ET tube connected to the wall O_2 outlet at 5–7 L/min. The test is discontinued if the patient's saturation falls below 90%, or 10 min are reached without any breathing efforts. A blood gas is done before the patient is connected to the ventilator to make sure that a pCO_2 of at least 8 kPa is reached. This means that there has been sufficient hypercarbia to stimulate the respiratory centre and that this centre is dysfunctional.

9
Paediatric Neurosurgery

CONTENTS

INTRODUCTION

This is a very large subject and the first part of this chapter is aimed at pointing out some of the main differences between paediatric and adult neurosurgery. The chapter then goes on to give to an overview of some of the developmental abnormalities which are specific to children. It should be emphasized, however, that this chapter is only a brief introduction to some of the aspects of paediatric neurosurgery. A fuller discussion is beyond the scope of this book.

DIFFERENCES BETWEEN PAEDIATRIC AND ADULT NEUROSURGERY

MALIGNANT AND VASCULAR PATHOLOGY

Cerebral tumours account for a much larger proportion of total malignancies in the paediatric population than in the adult population where bronchial and breast cancer far outstrip brain cancer. Children tend to adjust to their deficits and frequently only complain in the later stages; signs are often picked up by the parents even before their child complains. This is certainly true for visual field deficits where the children will continue without complaint and are only diagnosed because they constantly bump into objects. Children have the same spectrum of glial tumours as adults but also have juvenile pilocytic astrocytoma which is a Grade I astrocytoma and quite benign. It differs from other benign tumours in that it enhances quite brightly with contrast. Embryonic tumours and stem-cell tumours, such as the primitive neuroectodermal tumours and the disembrioplastic neuroepithelial tumours, are part of the childhood tumour spectrum. Embryonic tumours are usually found in the midline. In the posterior fossa the differential diagnoses for tumours are astrocytomas, medulloblastoma or ependymoma. Children are also more prone to developmental inclusion tumours, such as epidermoids and craniopharyngiomas. Brainstem gliomas are also much more common, and focal, slow-growing gliomas carry a much better prognosis than the diffuse pontine gliomas which present with an enlarged so-called 'fat pons'. Optic and hypothalamic gliomas are also more prevalent in the paediatric population. A spinal tumour in the adult would be more likely to be an ependymoma than it would be in a child; in children, gliomas of the spinal cord dominate, along with gangliogliomas.

Vascular pathology differs from that in adults, and children with SAH are most likely to have an underlying AVM rather than an aneurysm. The management of the SAH, and treatment of vascular abnormalities, follow the same principles as in adults.

ICU

The management of the paediatric patient in ICU is a topic on its own and falls outside the scope of this book. However, it is noteworthy that, in the management of raised ICP, hyperventilation in children is much more effective than it is in adults. Children do not have the degree of renal compensation that adults possess and that, in adults, tends to negate the good effects of hyperventilation. They also do not have the same degree of ischaemia-related problems that one sees in adults.

TRAUMA

In children, a minor or moderate head injury can sometimes be followed by malignant hyperaemia which causes severe brain swelling and can be quite refractory to treatment. Spinal trauma in children tends to incur ligamentous damage more than fractures and may result in SCIWORA (spinal cord injury without radiological abnormality). This is particularly true in the cervical spine. This is because children have relatively large head in comparison to the rest of their body, weak neck muscles, weak and lax ligaments, and horizontally-aligned facet joints.

DEVELOPMENTAL ABNORMALITIES

Abnormalities in neural tube formation are a large group of developmental abnormalities. Failure of closure during secondary neurulation leads to spinal dysraphism, whilst secondary reopening after closure leads to cranial dysraphism.

SPINAL DYSRAPHISM

There are a few general features of spinal dysraphisms. In occult lesions, there are frequently external stigmata of underlying dysraphism, such as a dimple, tuft of hair, or hyperpigmentation. There is usually some form of bony abnormality and spinal cord tethering is a frequent feature. A brief description of some of the more common abnormalities follows.

Open lesions

Myelomeningocoele

In this condition, the whole spinal cord is visible through a thin layer of arachnoid. As a result of spina bifida there is no soft tissue cover or bony cover, and the spinal cord is a flat, unrolled structure with the dorsal surface respresenting the area that would have formed the central canal. The arachnoid tears easily, and in such cases spinal fluid will leak out. It is imperative that babies with this condition are nursed on their tummies or sides, so as to stop damage to the neural placode; the neural tissue should be kept moist with a saline-soaked swab. These babies usually have associated abnormalities with hindbrain herniation and Chiari 2 malformation, hydrocephalus, and foot and other organ abnormalities. The amniotic fluid of the mother is toxic to neural tissue and babies will usually have a neurological deficit with sphincter dysfunction and variable level of motor and sensory deficit. The deficit depends on the level of the lesion, with thoracic and cervical lesions having higher levels of neurological compromise than those associated with lumbosacral lesions. It is imperative that these lesions are closed within the first day, or at most 2 days, to prevent infection and also to limit neurological damage. Most babies also need CSF diversion with a shunt. These patients will go on to undergo multiple orthopaedic procedures and frequently have a urinary bypass performed and a colostomy done. A proportion of these patients go on to have a fairly normal life depending on their IQ and the number of shunt revisions.

Meningocoele

The main feature is a fluid-filled sac on the posterior aspect of the spinal cord without any neural tissue therein. Closure is mandatory to prevent infection of the CSF.

Skin-covered lesions (occult lesions)

Spina bifida occulta

This is frequently diagnosed by chance in somebody undergoing lumbar X-rays for other reasons, or it can be part of another dysraphic state, like myelomeningocoel, meningocoel etc.

Lipomyelomeningocoele

This lesion is characterized by a lipoma over the lumbosacral spine, which is attached with a stalk through a bony defect to an intraspinal lipoma with associated spinal tethering and spinal root compression. Since the cauda equina is usually intertwined with the lipoma, this can be quite a daunting surgical prospect. There are three anatomical variants: (1) the dorsal type, which consists of a lipoma dorsal to the nerve roots; (2) the terminal type, which consists of a lipoma at the site of the filum; and (3) the transitional type, which consists of a lipoma lying in an intermediate position between dorsal and terminal types. Failure to decompress these lesions leads to progressive nerve root compression, with pain, paraesthesia, numbness and motor and sphincter dysfunction.

Meningocoele

This is the same as the meningocoele in open lesions, except that, in this case, the lesion is covered by skin. The urgency of surgical correction is obviated by the fact that the skin cover prevents infection of the CSF.

Anterior myelomeningocoel/meningocoele

This is a lesion where the dysraphism presents to the abdominal cavity and not the back, and is rapidly fatal if not diagnosed promptly and treated.

Spinal cord tethering

There is usually a small associated lipoma at the lower end of the filum, the filum is thickened to more than 2 mm, and the conus is below the level of the L2 vertebra due to tension on the developing cord from the tethered filum. Children with these lesions present, in their teenage years during the growth spurt, with radicular symptoms and the inability to flex forward due to an exacerbation of their symptoms. Loosening of the tethered cord is an option but carries a significant risk of root damage.

Diastematomyelia

In diastematomyelia there are duplications of the spinal cord, due to the interposition in the developing cord of a bony ridge or membrane. Spinal cords can be invested in a single dura or they can have duplication of the dura and separate coverings as well. Surgery to remove the bony ridge or membrane is done when there is nervous compression.

Dorsal dermal sinus

When neuroectoderm fails to separate from the superficial ectoderm, a sinus may remain. This may provide a route of infection and produce recurrent bacterial meningitis. Surgical correction with excision of the sinus is mandatory.

CRANIAL DYSRAPHISM

Encephalocoele

These are outpouchings of the brain with its covering through a cranial defect. The brain is usually atrophic and nonfunctional, and the prognosis depends on the amount of brain tissue present in the lesion. These lesions are divided into anterior and posterior encephalocoeles, and the anterior group are divided into basal (skull base), sincipital (midface) and frontal (frontal bone) lesions. The posterior lesions are divided into a supratorcular and an infratorcular group (the Torcula of Herophili is the confluence of the sinuses.) The basis of management is the resection of the protruded tissue and closure of the defect, with a team approach by the neurosurgeons, plastic and maxillofacial surgeons.

Craniofacial abnormalities

Combined facial, cranial and systemic abnormalities are found in these syndromes, with some of the most common being Apert's, Crouzon's and Pheiffer's syndromes. These are treated by a combined team approach as with the encephalocoeles described above.

Congenital hydrocephalus

This is usually diagnosed *in utero* in the modern era of imaging. Babies born with hydrocephalus may present with increased diameter of the head, the 'setting-sun' sign in cases of severe pressure (this is the paediatric equivalent of Parinaud's phenomenon: palsy of upward or downward gaze, dissociation of light and accommodation reflex, failure of convergence). The hydrocephalus is usually of the noncommunicating type and requires CSF diversion. Babies and children can, however, also develop communicating hydrocephalus secondary to intracranial infections and haemorrhages. The same principles apply as for adults, with the exception that the skull of babies and toddlers is more compliant since the anterior fontanel usually closes only at 18 months.

10
Basic Neurosurgical Procedures

CONTENTS

INTRODUCTION

During your time as a neurosurgical SHO you will have the opportunity to see a multitude of wonderful and dramatic operations. Unfortunately, you will be unlikely to get heavily involved in most of these at this stage of your training. However, there are certain procedures which are performed commonly enough to be classified as 'basic'. In this context 'basic' means that a junior trainee would be expected to be familiar with the principles of these procedures, rather than that the procedures are minor or easy. Familiarize yourself with these procedures by reading this chapter and make sure you see each being performed early in your job. You should then make every effort actually to perform these procedures, or at least part of them. Obviously, this is particularly important if you are planning a career in neurosurgery. Getting properly involved in these operations will also help you to enjoy the job better, even if you plan to be an orthopaedic or general surgeon.

The following is an account of the relevant procedures in which you should try to get involved. A large majority of out-of hours emergency operating will involve diversion of CSF flow (EVDs and shunts), evacuation of haematomas (CSDH, ASDH, EDH) and spinal decompression. These procedures will occur frequently enough during your on-calls for you to have ample opportunities to familiarize yourself with them.

CRANIAL PROCEDURES

SOME BASIC SURFACE ANATOMY

The principles of opening the cranium are the same as for any other body cavity. You need to have an appreciation of the basic surface anatomy and the relationship to deeper structures, so that you can avoid unnecessary complications. When incising the scalp it is essential to appreciate where scalp vessels run, so that they can be preserved. The integrity of a scalp flap is dependent on a good blood supply, and although individual vessels might be sacrificed without too much harm, to minimize the risk of necrosis no vessels should be sacrificed.

You will, of course, recall from your anatomy days that there are six arteries on each side of the head which supply the scalp. The anterior two arteries are branches of the internal carotid artery (cranial portion, as this artery has no branches in the neck): supratrochlear and supraorbital arteries. The other four arteries are branches of the external carotid artery: superficial temporal artery; posterior auricular artery; and occipital artery. There are plentiful anastamoses between these arteries but there is a danger of isolating a flap from its blood supply by cutting across them incautiously. Neurosurgical scalp flaps are, therefore, made based upon these arteries. Perhaps the branch most relevant to the junior trainee is the superficial temporal artery, the pulsation of which can be palpated just in front of the tragus. When making the incision for the trauma craniotomy described below, it is prudent to palpate for this artery and begin your incision posterior to it. Another rule to adhere to is to make sure that the bottom half of the flap is never less than half the length of the top edge.

The nerve supply of the scalp itself is of less concern to the neurosurgeon. A small area of scalp anaesthesia is a small price to pay for the evacuation of a life-threatening haematoma. However, the temporal branch of the facial nerve can be damaged by an injudiciously placed incision, and this will result in a noticeable deficit later on. The temporal branch of the facial nerve passes from within the substance of the parotid gland and crosses above the zygomatic arch about 1 inch in front of the tragus. Incisions in the zygomatic area are, therefore, kept less than 1/2 inch anterior to the tragus and above the zygomatic arch so as to avoid damage to this nerve.

For the purposes of the procedures described here, the next most important structures to be aware of are the dural venous sinuses and the motor strip. Provided that burr-holes are placed well away from these areas the risks will be kept to a minimum. The sagittal sinus runs in the midline and so burrs are cut over 2.5 cm from the midline. It is important, when draping patients, to make sure that you can still confidently identify the midline.

Other sinuses, such as the lateral sinus, should be well away from your drill as you should not be cutting near the posterior fossa. The motor cortex is located 4–5 cm behind the coronal suture which, with practice on yourself, should be easily palpable through the scalp. Alternatively, the position of the superior aspect of the motor cortex can be estimated by following a vertical line up through the external auditory meatus. An oft-quoted method is to use a tape measure (or piece of string that can be halved by folding) to find the mid point of the arc extending from nasion to inion (external occipital protruberance): the motor cortex is 2 cm posterior to this point. Figure 32 summarizes these three methods for estimating the position of the motor strip. The transverse sinus can be marked out by drawing a line from the tragus to the external occipital protuberance.

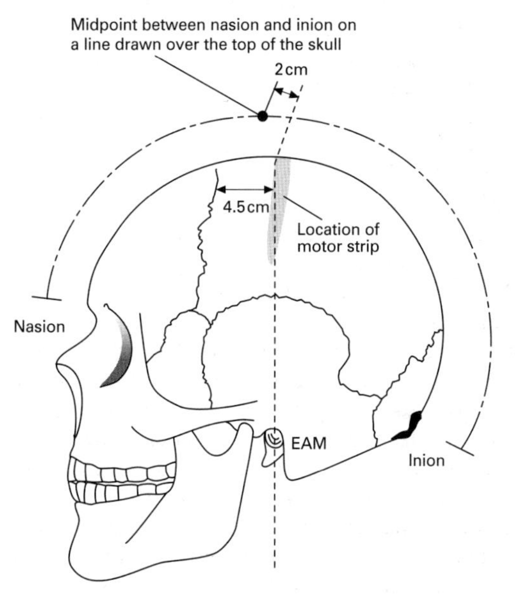

Figure 32. Diagram summarizing three methods of estimating the position of the motor strip in relation to the skull. EAM = external auditory meatus.

INSERTION OF AN ICP BOLT

Insertion of ICP bolts may be done in the ICU to monitor the ICP in patients with diffuse head injury. If a patient goes to theatre, then insertion of ICP-monitoring devices is ideally performed at the time of surgery. If performed in the ICU, it is imperative that the procedure is carried out in as sterile a manner as possible.

Ideally, the surgeon will be positioned at the head of the patient, who is lying supine. Identify, shave, and mark Kocher's point, which is 1 cm anterior to the coronal suture in the midpupillary line, which is about 2.5 cm from the midline (see Figure 33). After cleaning the area and injecting some

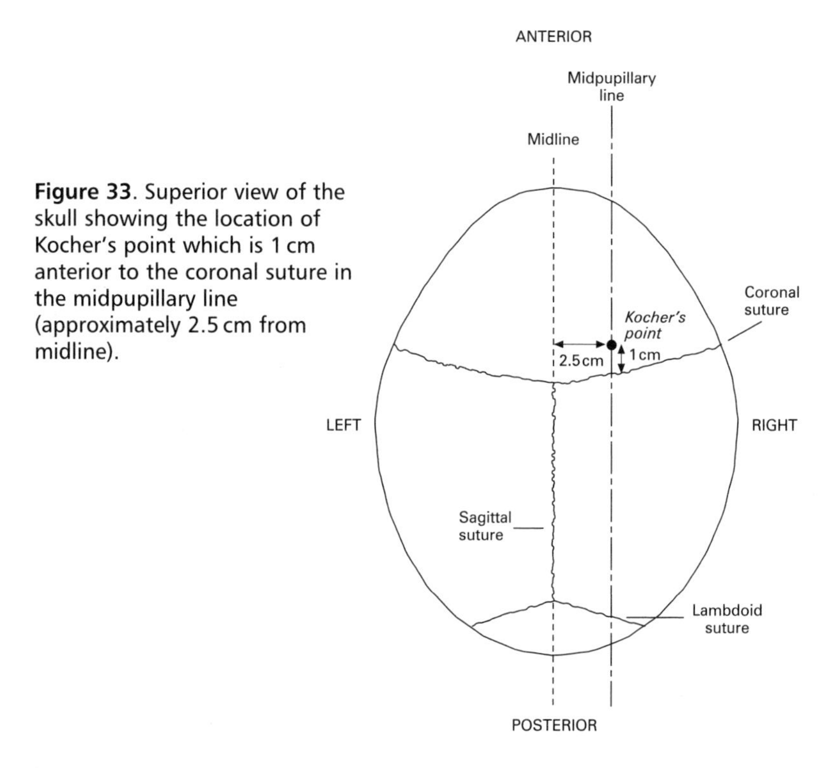

Figure 33. Superior view of the skull showing the location of Kocher's point which is 1 cm anterior to the coronal suture in the midpupillary line (approximately 2.5 cm from midline).

local anaesthetic (e.g., 2 ml lignocaine with adrenaline) make a small vertical stab incision (no more than 0.5 cm long) with a small blade, down to the skull. A twist drill is used to penetrate the skull. There should be a spur or shoulder on the drill to prevent plunging it into the brain. Once the skull has been breached, a small cylindrical tap is screwed into the hole to allow for passage of the ICP catheter. It is advisable to calibrate the ICP monitor at this point before opening the dura. The exact procedure for calibration will differ between makes of machine, and the ICU staff will usually be familiar with the one they keep in stock (it usually involves obtaining a zero reading whilst the monitor wire is in sterile water and writing down a reference number). The dura is opened by pricking it with a pin placed down the cylindrical tap. The pin will be provided by the manufacturer and will usually have a right angle on it to prevent its going too far or being lost inside the cranium. A small back-flow of CSF is usually seen as the pin passes through the dura. The ICP monitor wire can now be passed down the tap (it should not exceed the inner surface of the cranium by more than 0.5 cm) and then screwed securely. Before attaching the ICP monitor wire to the monitor, make sure that it is securely fastened so as to reduce the chances of its being pulled out.

BURR-HOLE DRAINAGE OF A CHRONIC SUBDURAL HAEMATOMA

The drainage of a subdural haematoma can usually be achieved through one or two burr-holes. Two may be helpful as this allows the washing of saline from one burr-hole through to the next. The location of the burr-holes will depend upon the location of the haematoma as determined by CT scan. However, the general principle is that burr-holes should be located along the same line as the incision of a trauma flap, so that, if there are any problems, it is relatively easy to proceed to a trauma craniotomy. The procedure can be performed under local anaesthetic but until you are more experienced, and unless the patient is likely to tolerate the procedure awake, it is best done under general anaesthetic. The patient is positioned supine on the operating table with the head placed on a ring. Check the side of the haematoma on the scan at this point and double check with a colleague. For burr-holes, the head can be kept straight or slightly angled to the side contralateral to the haematoma. It should be borne in mind that, if it is necessary to proceed to craniotomy, the head will need to be rotated further laterally (see below). Once the head is positioned, the hair can be shaved and the skin incisions marked out (aprox. 2–3 cm in length). The incisions should be placed along the line of an appropriate craniotomy such as the question-mark-shaped temporoparietal craniotomy described below. Ensure that your incisions are located so that the burr-holes will overlie the subdural haematoma. It is essential, therefore, to look at the scan again and decide the height of the haematoma in the cranium and its anteroposterior extent. Prep and drape the patient so that you can still locate the midline and can feel relevant landmarks, such as the glabella and external auditory meatus. Inform the anaesthetist, and infiltrate local anaesthetic with adrenaline into the sites of your incision. Before picking up the scalpel check the side one more time. If the site of your incision is above the superficial temporal line (which it most probably will be) you will be able to cut directly through skin down to bone. Use the handle of the knife, or the handle of a periosteal elevator, to push the periosteum away from the skull. If you are using two burr-holes, prepare the second site before drilling. Insert a self-retainer to hold the wound open and expose the skull. You will find that the self-retainer will control most bleeding points from the scalp edges, but use bipolar diathermy to control any obvious bleeders. You are now ready to use the drill. Make sure that you are comfortable and hold the drill in both hands. Make sure that the patient's head is well supported by your assistant. You will be taught how to use the drill, but the following points must always be remembered: apply a constant firm pressure but without leaning your body-weight on the drill; the drill will stop automatically once the cranium is breached and when it does take your foot off the drill pedal (and not before, as the clutch will disengage and it will not be possible to start it again.) and withdraw the drill. Never restart the drill in the burr-hole once the drill has stopped. You should now be able to see dura and, if the burr-hole is properly located, you will see the dark blue of the subdural haematoma underneath. Control any bleeding from the bone with bone wax, and remove any fragments of remaining bone with a blunt hook and fine-toothed forceps. Now use the diathermy to scorch the whole area of exposed dura. Open the dura by making a cruciate incision with an appropriately sized knife and sharp hook. It is safest to make a small incision to begin and then use the hook to lift the dura towards you. Once the dura has been incised in this way there will be four triangular leaves of dura. Shrink these back to the bone by grasping them with the bipolar and coagulating them. If the membranes around the CSDH have not burst by this point then scorch it with the bipolar and open it with a blunt instrument like a Macdonald. Alternatively, hold the bipolar tips close together and advance them into the membrane and allow them to open up (again, scorch the membranes as you advance). Once through, you will find that the dark brown fluid that constitutes a CSDH will drain out. Wash the subdural space through carefully with saline. Some surgeons insert soft catheters into the subdural space to wash it out, but it is important to avoid damage to the brain and using only a syringe can be a safer option in the junior surgeon's hands. You will see the surface of the brain and you should try to allow it to expand towards the cranium. This may happen spontaneously or you might ask the anaesthetist to induce a Valsalva manoeuvre to speed things up. Before closing the wounds ensure that you have filled any gaps between the brain and skull as much as possible with saline. You may either leave the burr-holes empty or fill them with Surgicel™, Spongistan™ or beeswax. Close the scalp with 2/0 or 3/0 Vicryl™ interrupted to the galea, and either clips or 3/0 nylon to the skin.

FRONTOTEMPOROPARIETAL TRAUMA CRANIOTOMY (DRAINAGE OF ASDH AND EDH)

The reason for describing this craniotomy is that the most common site for an ASDH is the surface of the frontotemporoparietal cortex. Also, this incision can be used to evacuate an EDH which has formed in the classic temporal location due to bleeding from the middle meningeal artery.

The patient is positioned supine, with the head rotated to the side contralateral to the clot. The idea is to position the patient such that there will be optimal view under all edges of the craniotomy. Generally speaking, you should aim to have the side of the head as horizontal as possible. This is facilitated by the placement of sand bags under the ipsilateral shoulder. The head is best fixed with a three-point head fixator.

Shave the side of the head affected, all the way to the midline. Mark out a question-mark shaped incision which begins at the zygomatic arch no more than a finger's breadth in front of the tragus. Remember to palpate for the superficial temporal artery and avoid it. The line of the incision is a curve back around the top of the ear and then a curve towards the midline. From here it runs parallel to the midline anteriorly to the hairline (see Figure 34). Prep and drape the patient.

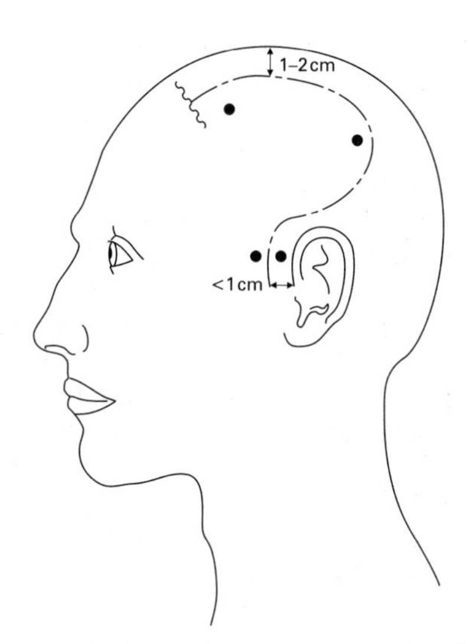

Figure 34. Diagram showing the location of a typical skin incision for a frontotemporoparietal craniotomy. Note that the location of four burr-holes is also shown: one frontal; one parietal; and two temporal. It is important to place the two temporal burr-holes low down in order to decompress temporal extradural haematomas.

Make an incision through the scalp along the line described above. This is a large incision and bleeding needs to be adequately controlled. This is achieved by direct pressure either side of the incision with the fingers on mastoid swabs. After every 5 cm or so of incision apply Raney scalp clips over the scalp edges to include the mastoid swabs. This should be an efficient, smooth process so as not to delay proceeding to the life-saving part of the operation. Part of your incision may take you directly down to bone but in the temporal area it will overlie the temporalis muscle. You will need to sweep the scalp forward over the surface of the muscle using a wet swab and the back of the scalpel blade to expose the muscle. Wrap the scalp flap in a wet swab and anchor it forward out of the way with rubber bands.

Cut through the temporalis muscle down to bone with the monopolar diathermy. The line of incision is just inside your skin incision in an inverted 'U' shape. Remember that, when you come to use the craniotome, you need to be about 3 cm from the midline so as to stay away from the sagittal sinus. Leave the lowermost neck of temporalis intact. Sweep the periosteum clear with the periosteal elevators along the line of the incision.

Place four burr-holes: one temporal; one at the pterion; one frontal; and one parietal. Connect the burr-holes with the craniotome except for the temporal and pterional ones. This will leave a bridge of bone inferiorly which will need to be broken when the bone flap is turned. Use bone elevators to lift the bone flap gently away from the dura, taking care not to tear it. Once you can safely get your fingers under the bone gently break the inferior bone edge. There is now a bone flap that opens out like a trap door which is hinged on the temporalis muscle; this is known as an osteoplastic flap.

You are now left with either of two situations, depending on the indication for the operation. You will see either a bright red EDH overlying the dura or a dark blue ASDH underneath the dura. In the case of an EDH, you have already performed the life saving procedure by opening the bone. There remains only to evacuate the haematoma by sucking away at it, and then placing dural hitch stitches to attach the dura to the edges of the craniotomy. This is to prevent the EDH from reaccumulating. Use a non-cutting needle and 3/0 Vicryl, taking care not to tear the dura or cause subdural bleeding by making sure that the needle passes only through the outer layer of the dura. It can be useful to slip a single layer of Surgicel between the dura and the bone to help haemostasis. When sucking away the haematoma, identify and control any bleeding points. Look under the edges of the craniotomy and remove any clots found. In the case of a subdural haematoma it is necessary to incise the dura to evacuate the underlying clot. Beware opening the dura too widely as the brain may swell and herniate out of your incision, risking laceration on the sharp dural edges. This is true for cases where it is obvious from the CT scan that there is a lot of brain swelling and mass effect from the haematoma, and in these cases it is safer simply to fenestrate the dura with small slit lacerations and suck out the clot gently. This allows clot evacuation while minimizing brain herniation.

The bone flap can be replaced and either fixed back with screws or bioplates, or allowed to ride free. Riding free may help control the ICP postoperatively. The scalp is closed with 2/0 or 3/0 Vicryl to the galea, and clips to the skin. This is a large flap and so a drain may be needed. When removing the Raney's ensure that you take care to diathermy any bleeding points as there can be profuse bleeding at this stage.

In the very acute situation, especially with an EDH, only the lower part of this exposure need be used. For example, in the case of a temporal EDH the first 5 cm or so of the incision can be made and the temporalis incised down to bone. A self-retainer is inserted and a temporal burr-hole made. This can be enlarged quickly using bone-clippers or rongeurs. This allows for extremely rapid decompression of the clot and can be life-saving.

INSERTION OF AN EVD

Insertion of a catheter into the frontal horn of the lateral ventricle is a lifesaving procedure in acute hydrocephalus and familiarity with the technique is essential. The patient is positioned supine with the head secured either on a ring or with a foam cushion. If the head is kept in the neutral position it is easier to coordinate catheter trajectory later on. Shave the right frontal area (the nondominant side is usual for catheter placement, unless there is a contraindication, e.g., underlying lesion). Identify and mark Kocher's point which is 1 cm anterior to the coronal suture in the midpupillary line (aprox. 2.5 cm from midline). This is the point at which the burr-hole will be made and the catheter inserted. Mark out a 2–3 cm incision centred on this point in a sagittal plane. Incise the scalp and fashion a burr-hole as described above. In this instance the dura does not need to be opened widely but just sufficient to allow passage of the catheter. Scorch the pial covering of the cortex with the bipolar diathermy and use the tip of a sharp blade to ensure that it has been breached. The next step is the most difficult part – placement of the catheter into the frontal horn of the lateral ventricle. There are numerous stereotactic methods described in the books and each is slightly different. The key is to have one method in mind, learn it and stick to it. Basically, if you pass the catheter perpendicular to the surface of the skull to a depth of 5 cm (less in presence of hydrocephalus) you will enter the frontal horn of the lateral ventricle. There are 5 cm and 10 cm markings on ventricular catheters. To help you ensure that the catheter is perpendicular you can check your position in the coronal and sagittal planes. In the coronal plane the catheter should be pointing towards the medial canthal line of the ipsilateral eye. In the sagittal plane the catheter should be pointing towards the external auditory meatus, or just anterior to it. When the catheter enters the ventricle you should feel a subtle 'give' and when the trocar is withdrawn you will drain CSF. Now advance the catheter with the trocar withdrawn. At this point it is imperative not to let the catheter move in relation to the skull. Hold the catheter with a pair of non-toothed forceps held flush to the skull while you tunnel the distal end of the catheter under the scalp to an exit point a few centimetres away from the skin wound. You would be well advised to secure the catheter in place with a few overlying sutures before closing the scalp incision. Attach your extraventricular drainage system and set it to a fixed setting, e.g., 10 cmH_2O. Close the scalp incision, taking care not to perforate the drain with your needle. Ensure that you secure the drain with a further series of sutures, as EVDs have a tendency to 'fall out' when patients are transferred.

INSERTION OF A VENTRICULOPERITONEAL SHUNT (OCCIPTAL CATHETER)

The patient is supine with a sand bag under the ipsilateral shoulder to allow good rotation of the head away from the site of insertion. The aim is to position the patient so as to provide as straight a line as possible from the occipital site of insertion distally across the neck and thorax to the abdominal site of insertion. Mark out the following: (1) the site of the occipital burr-hole (6 cm superior to the external occipital protruberance and 3 cm from the midline); (2) an incision around the burr-hole so that the incision does not lie over the top of the shunt site; (3) an abdominal incision. Prep the whole area all the way from head to abdomen. Drape to expose the whole shunt path. It may be necessary to staple drapes in the neck area to ensure that they are flush with the skin. Stop, and go through in your mind the sequence of events:

1. Open scalp and drill burr-hole – do not open dura.
2. Open abdomen – clip, but do not open peritoneum.
3. Tunnel, and pass distal catheter (and valve, if attached to catheter).
4. Open dura and pass proximal catheter.
5. Connect proximal catheter to valve (in the case of separate shunt-valve kits).
6. Check CSF flow through shunt.
7. Open peritoneum and pass distal catheter.
8. Close wounds.

Before proceeding, prepare the shunt by taking it out of its packaging and priming and soaking it in gentamicin. Make a curved scalp incision around the planned site of the burr-hole. The site of the burrhole is 6 cm up from the inion (external occipital protruberance) and 3 cm lateral to the midline. Take great care with haemostasis at this stage (you can use monopolar once you are through the skin if you prefer). It is useful to have forceps and mastoid swabs in one hand and diathermy in the other. Remember that water runs down-hill, so start at the top of the wound and work down, otherwise your view will always be obscured by bleeders higher up. Also, cut vessels have two ends so always check the other side of the wound if you find a big bleeder on one side. A useful tip is to develop scalp layers so that the aponeurosis can be separated and flipped back. This can be sutured over the proximal catheter later, adding strength to the proximal catheter.

Use scissors to develop a plane distally for receipt of valve and catheter: place the scissors in closed, then open them up and withdraw. Make the burr-hole. Cover the proximal wound with Betadine-soaked swabs. Take care never to touch the edges of wounds.

Now go to the abdomen and open it up. This is similar to an appendix incision, except that it is in the upper part of the abdomen: knife to skin; Langenbecks through fat; scissors through muscle; clips to peritoneum (do not open yet). Leave the clips on the peritoneum and cover the wound with Betadine-soaked swabs.

You are now ready to tunnel and pass the distal shunt. It is advisable to change gloves at this stage. Place clean swabs over the abdomen so that the shunt end can remain as sterile as possible once passed. It is academic whether you tunnel in a distal-to-proximal direction or vice versa. Bend the guide to the correct shape first (use the surface of the patient as a guide). Take care to advance over the clavicle and not to burrow into the neck. Remove the central trocar and pass the shunt through.

Now open the dura with diathermy in the centre of the burr-hole and pass the tip of the knife through. Use diathermy to extend the hole slightly and then buzz the surface of the brain only slightly. Pass the proximal catheter directed towards the glabella to a depth of 4 cm (or check the distance on the scan) and feel for entry into the ventricle. Remove the trocar to check for CSF flow and advance the catheter. Place the bulldog clip on the catheter to control the CSF flow and cut the catheter to the length required (i.e., almost flush with the skull – be careful not to lose the proximal catheter inside the cranium at this stage!).

Connect the two parts of the shunt system and tie securely with 2/0 Vicryl. Take care not to pull the proximal catheter out at this stage. Remove the bulldog clip and check for CSF flow distally; aspirate if necessary.

Close the head wound with 2/0 or 3/0 Vicryl and clips to skin (it is best to use clips, as needles risk perforating the shunt). Remember that, if you developed the scalp layers, the aponeurosis can be flapped over the proximal catheter for extra protection.

Open the peritoneum by holding up the attached clips and checking with thumb and forefinger for the bowel before opening with the scissors. Introduce the distal end of the shunt into the peritoneal cavity. There is no need to suture the peritoneum unless you have made more than a very tiny incision. Close the aponeuroses and muscle with 3/0 Vicryl and use subcutaneous Vicryl to skin.

SPINAL PROCEDURES

LUMBAR PUNCTURE

The patient is positioned on their side with their knees curled up towards the chest. The back, straight or flexed anteriorly, should be close to the edge of the bed. As the spinal cord ends at L1/2 (continuing as the cauda equina below) the ideal intervertebral space to aim for is L4/5. This can be identified easily, as the highest point of the iliac crest is located on a level with the spinous process of the fourth lumbar vertebra. Feel for the space between the L4 and L5 spinous processes and mark the spot. It is helpful to ensure that, when the area has been cleaned and draped, it is possible to feel the iliac crest without contaminating the hands: this allows the level to be rechecked. Local anaesthetic is injected down to bone and below the skin. The spinal needle is advanced slowly in the midline in the L4/5 interspace in a slightly rostral orientation. The needle will be felt to 'give' when the dura is breached, and a backflash of CSF will be seen when the trocar is withdrawn. The central trocar should now be removed and a manometer attached to measure the opening pressure (this should always be done). A three-way tap attached between the manometer and spinal needle will allow CSF from the manometer to be taken for analysis. If the L4/5 interspace is not encountered the first time then further attempts can be made with the same needle provided that the tip is not withdrawn from the skin between passes. Always make sure that the patient is as comfortable as possible and enquire expressly about nerve root pain in the legs (withdraw the needle if pain is felt).

LUMBAR DRAIN PLACEMENT

The procedure to place a lumbar drain is similar to that for a lumbar puncture, except that a larger needle is used which has an angled opening at the tip. This allows a drain to be inserted and guided into the vertebral canal. Care should be taken to orientate the bevel so that the sharp cutting-edge runs parallel to the nerve roots. This reduces the risk of severing the root on insertion. Once in the canal, the needle can be rotated 90° to direct the passage of the drain into the canal.

LAMINECTOMY

The most common laminectomies that are encountered are lumbar and cervical, although thoracic laminectomies will also be seen. The positioning and techniques will differ for each, but the basic principles are the same for all three regions. Patients undergoing cervical laminectomy will be prone, and their heads will be fixed firmly, e.g., with a Mayfield. The position is described as the concorde position as the neck is in flexion. It is important to ensure that the face of the patient is not pressing on anything that may cause injury and that the anaesthetist is happy with the airway. In patients undergoing lumbar laminectomy it is important to ensure that the abdomen is not under any pressure, as this would result in increased venous pressure and excessive bleeding in the surgical field. Pressure can be reduced with the use of a pillow under the pelvis and one higher up at the level of the thorax.

There are several ways of determining the spinal level for the laminectomy. One way is to use spinal needles and the image intensifier. However, it may be better to prep and drape the patient beforehand to minimize the risk of infection. Once the levels have been marked, an appropriate midline incision can be marked out. After infiltration of local anaesthetic, a midline incision is made down to the spinous processes. If the incision is truly in the midline then there will be minimal damage to the paravertebral muscles.

The muscles are detached from the spinous processes with cutting diathermy. Care should be taken at the depths of the wound such that the diathermy is not pushed through the interspinous spaces into the spinal canal. The muscle is then stripped away from the laminae with a retractor and mastoid swabs. The rectangular mastoids are inserted vertically into the wound parallel to the spinous processes. The cob is then used to sweep the mastoids laterally out along the laminae, thus lifting the paravertebral muscles away from the bone. A self-retaining retractor system can now be used to hold the wound open. The spinous processes and the laminae should now be clearly visible. It may be necessary to take some time to clean any remaining tissue from the bone. The spinal level should be checked again at this point, using artery clips as markers and visualising with the image intensifier.

The relevant spinous processes are removed by using a Horsley's (single action rangeurs) or bone shears to break them away from the laminae. The Horsley's can be used in 'Herring bone' fashion to remove the remaining bases of the spinous processes.

The spinal canal is opened with a small 1–2 mm vertical punch carefully placed under the edge of the laminae. The first bites should be done with caution and the punch should never be forced into a space. If there is any doubt, probe carefully with a blunt instrument. With diligence and persistence an opening will eventually be made and the spinal canal can be opened. The opening can be increased gradually by taking bites from alternate sides and working up the canal (using a larger 3–5 mm punch, provided that it fits). Care is taken not to puncture the dura or to take bites out of the nerve roots. As a general rule, work upwards when removing bone and downwards when removing ligamentum. Knowledge of the anatomy of the spinal cord and vertebral canal is essential for this to be done safely. Remember: unless the surgeon knows which parts of the procedure are risky, it is not safe to proceed.

The canal is opened over a given number of predetermined vertebral levels. If the procedure is for decompression of a stenosis, then the canal is widened until the dura is free and not compressed. Otherwise the canal is opened only so far as is required, e.g., for the removal of an extradural abscess or tumour.

The wound is closed with several layers of deep Vicryl suture. The surgeon's preference will determine the skin suture.

11

The Operative Microscope

The better we see, the more we know. The better we know, the more we see.

Gazi Yasargil

CONTENTS

HISTORICAL PERSPECTIVE

There are two events that stand out as being integral to the advancement of modern surgery: the introduction of anaesthesia by Morton and Simpson in the 1840s; and the discovery of antisepsis by Lister in the 1860s. In neurosurgery, perhaps the most significant factor to have produced advances has been the introduction of the surgical microscope.

Almost 200 years before Lister's antisepsis, Anton van Leeuwenhoek from Holland first observed the microorganisms responsible for infection, when he described the 'animalicules' he saw down his microscope. The development of the microscope, however, was the combination of a number of factors. Lenses were almost certainly known to man over 2000 years ago. Indeed, references to magnifying glasses appear in the writings of the Roman philosopher, Pliny, in the first century AD. The development of glass lenses led to the making of spectacles, and it was the Dutch spectacle makers, Zaccharias and Hans Janssen (father and son), who first experimented with several lenses in a tube, thus building the first compound microscope (it was these experiments that stimulated Galileo to work out the principles of lenses and subsequently to build the first telescope in 1609). Anton von Leeuwenhoek and Robert Hooke may rightly be called the fathers of microscopy, having refined the first microscopes and used them to make great scientific discoveries: it was Hooke who first described the term 'cell'.

The scientific advances that stem from microscopy have had a huge impact on medicine and, therefore, on surgery. However, it was not until the 20th century that the microscope was brought into the operating theatre and had a direct impact on operative technique. Successful collaborations between science and industry in the late 19th and early 20th century undoubtly laid the foundations for the development of microsurgery, as the field of optics was propelled forward. The industrial pioneer, Dr Carl Friedrich Zeiss, collaborated with Ernst Abbe of the University of Jena to develop theories of microscopic imaging and make optics technology widely available. Before the end of the 19th century, the company founded by Carl Zeiss had introduced the use of crystal to industrial optics. The growth in the optics industry in the first half of the 20th century meant that, in the late 1950s and early 1960s, a number of surgical specialties were able to introduce microscopes into their operative practice. The two fields in which the operating microscope first had an impact were vascular and plastic surgery. The degrees of magnification now available allowed for anastamosis of increasingly smaller surgical targets. Harry Buncke, in 1964, reported the successful transplantation of a rabbit ear in which he reattached the amputated part using vessels less than 1 mm in diameter.

Almost simultaneously, a number of neurosurgeons became interested in applying this powerful new tool to their own practice. In 1965, Gazi Yasargil, a native of Turkey, who had trained in Switzerland, undertook a period of work at the University of Vermont in the United States and visited plastic and vascular laboratories throughout the country to learn about the use of the microscope in surgery. Yasargil's work led to the development of new microsurgical techniques, particularly in the field of aneurysm surgery. Around the same time, Jules Hardy introduced a Zeiss OPM1 surgical microscope into the field of pituitary surgery in Montreal. The improvements in technique and greater surgical exposure led Hardy to formulate the idea that microadenomas were separable from normal pituitary tissue, and this led to further developments in the treatment of hypersecreting pituitary disorders. The operating microscope required the development of specialized microsurgical instruments and the establishment of the new field of microsurgical anatomy. Albert Rhoton of the University of Florida has employed the microscope over many years to develop the discipline of microsurgical anatomy.

Yasargil has described microneurosurgery as a field with two arms. On the one hand there is the equipment: the microscopes and the particularly delicate and specialized instruments. On the other hand is the skill of the neurosurgeon, who has to develop new indirect eye–hand interactions. The combination of stereoscopic magnification and illumination of deep structures in the CNS enables the surgeon to minimize retractive manoeuvres, preserve vital structures, and undertake delicate procedures. The following description introduces the operating microscope as it is used in neurosurgery. It is hoped that this brief introduction to the most influential neurosurgical instrument will help demystify it and allow the new trainee to make the best use of it early on.

COMPONENTS OF THE OPERATING MICROSCOPE

The first step in mastering the use of the operative microscope is to familiarize yourself with the various parts of the apparatus. Most operating microscopes consist of a base with light source from which an arm carrying the lens system and controls will extend. The arm will usually have more than one set of viewing eyepieces so that both the surgeon and assistant can view simultaneously. This is made possible by a beam-splitter – a semi-translucent mirror that splits a portion of the beam in a different direction while the main beam continues to the main viewer. In addition, there will be a connection to a monitor so that other members of the team – in particular the scrub nurse, anaesthetist, and attendant trainees – can follow the operation. It is worth taking the time to familiarize yourself with the various components of the microscope in your own unit. Make sure you can identify the following features (see Figure 35).

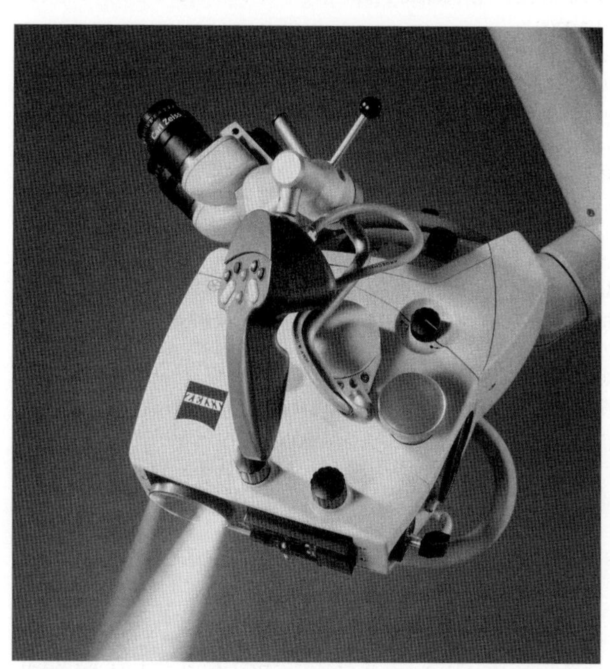

Figure 35. The eyepieces and controls of a Carl Zeiss operating microscope.

EYEPIECES

These are individually adjustable and provide a source of crude focusing. You should set the eyepiece dioptre scale to zero if you have normal vision or wear glasses that correct your vision. However, should you wish to discard your glasses during the operation you can adjust the eye pieces accordingly. It is important to recognize, though, that the eyepieces do not correct astigmatism.

BINOCULAR TUBE

The eyepieces are mounted on a binocular tube which rotates and can, therefore, be manoeuvred so that the surgeon remains in a comfortable position while operating. It is also possible to adjust the interpupillary distance: it is essential to adjust this so that both eyes are looking down the microscope, otherwise depth perception will be compromised.

MAGNIFICATION ADJUSTER

Modern operative microscopes have a fully motorized system (with manual backup) to adjust magnification (zoom) and focus. The magnification system is based on three pairs of lenses: one pair is fixed and the other two move up and down. In manual microscopes there may also be an objective lens which determines the working distance between the microscope and the operative field. In motorized magnification systems, however, the objective lens is incorporated in the magnification adjuster.

BASE WITH LIGHT SOURCE

The microscope will usually have a floor base but some units will have a ceiling mount. Due to the weight of the arm, the microscope is extremely finely balanced on the base. This needs to be checked before each operating session and you will hear theatre staff referring to 'balancing the microscope'. Whilst operating, it is obviously essential to be able to reposition the microscope over the operative field without upsetting the balance. This is made possible by the incorporation of electromagnetic coupling which can be released briefly by hand, foot, or mouth controls. The light source is located in the base and light is transmitted *via* a coaxial cable to the head of the microscope.

CONTROL PANEL

Control panels will vary between microscopes but are invariably located within easy reach of the surgeon. They are mostly straightforward, with zoom and focus controls and a button to release the lock on the microscope so that it can be repositioned.

PREPARING THE MICROSCOPE FOR USE

SETUP

Before beginning any operation the surgeon should be happy with the setup of the microscope. This includes the position of both sets of viewing

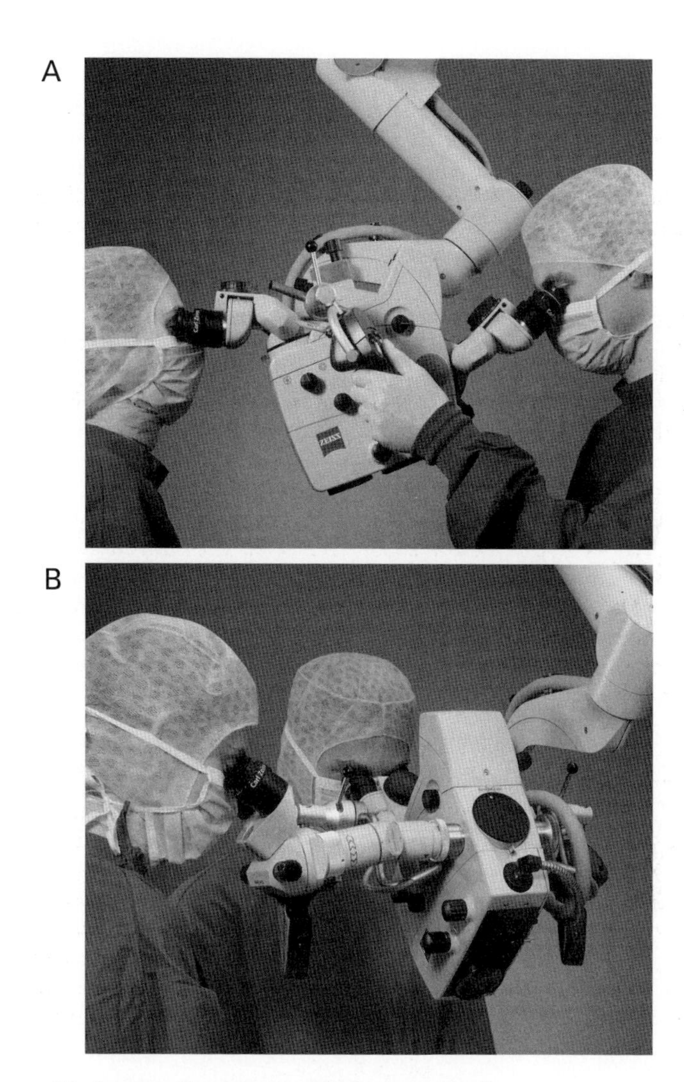

Figure 36. An operating neurosurgical microscope in:
(A) head-to-head configuration; and (B) side-on configuration.

eyepieces with respect to one another, as this will determine where the assistant stands. It is necessary to consider the site of the operation and where the best place for the assistant will be, e.g., in lumbar spine operations with a prone patient the eyepieces will face one another (head-to-head configuration) so that the assistant can be on the opposite side of the patient to the surgeon, but in cranial surgery it may be better to have the eye pieces at 90∫ to one another (side-on configuration). Figure 36 shows head-to-head and side-on configurations. Once the eyepieces are set correctly the surgeon should check the rest of the set-up. The following is a useful check-list:

1. Eyepieces – set the interpupillary distance to suit your eyes. Then set the eyepieces to 0 dioptres. If you are wearing glasses, fold down the rubber eye cups to prevent scratching the lenses of your glasses.
2. Magnification – set the microscope to the lowest magnification (usually ×0.5). The focus should be set in the middle of its travel.
3. Switch on the illumination.
4. Focus the microscope on a suitable object, e.g., a cross drawn on a piece of paper. If necessary, adjust the individual eyepieces to make the focus perfect.
5. Take an instrument in your hand and manipulate it under the microscope, making sure that you are comfortable with the settings.
6. Make sure that the assistant's microscope is set up properly. Ideally, the assistant needs to adjust his/her eyepieces.

DRAPING

Draping is performed by the nursing staff and is a sterile procedure whereby a sterile plastic drape is used to cover the microscope. The drape is specially designed and has pouches to incorporate the eyepieces and control handles of the microscope. There will usually be detachable plastic coverings over the eyepieces, and these need to be removed to allow clear viewing. Remember that, once the coverings have been removed, the area around the eyepieces will be unsterile. You will need to resist the temptation to handle the eyepieces during the operation.

POSITIONING

Most procedures will not require the microscope for the initial exposure. Microscopes on a base will, therefore, need to be brought closer to the operating table when they are required. Forethought will be needed so that space is left for them. Once in position they should be accessible without obstructing other vital components of the operating theatre. Figure 37 shows a microscope positioned and in use.

USING THE MICROSCOPE

The main functions of the operating microscope are to magnify and to illuminate the operative field. If you are unable to see because the structures are too small or the field is too dark, then use of the microscope is indicated. Unless the exposure is poor, or you are unfortunate enough to

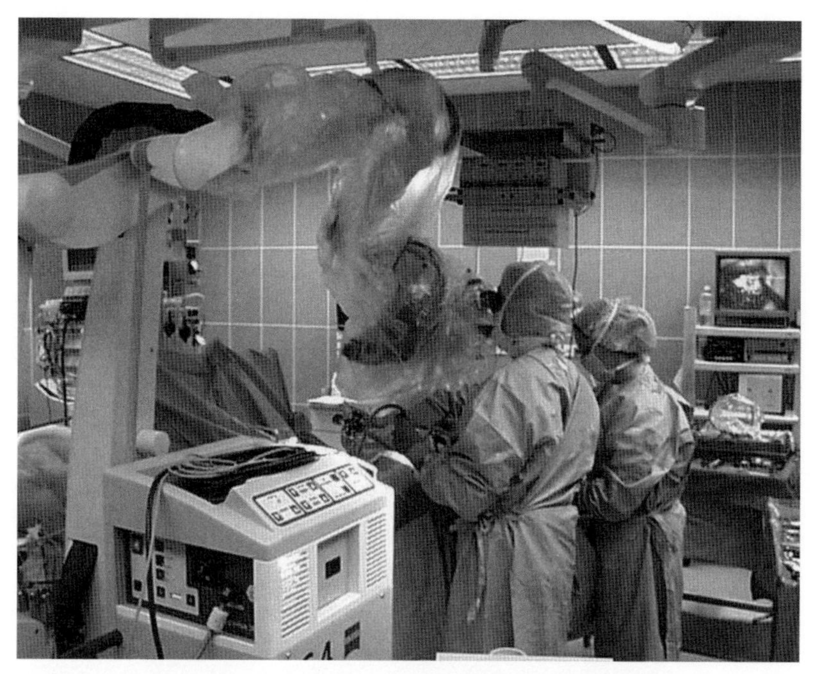

Figure 37. An operating neurosurgical microscope draped and in use.

have excessive bleeding in the operative field, then a poor view should never be a problem in neurosurgery. In order to achieve the dual objectives of magnification and illumination, the microscope needs to be positioned correctly.

Remember that, when operating without the microscope, the surgeon will need to move their head to view all parts of the operative field. The same principle applies to the microscope and frequent adjustments are necessary to look into all the corners of the operative field. In addition, there needs to be enough space between the field and the microscope to allow insertion and manipulation of instruments. The handling of instruments with indirect hand–eye coordination is a skill that can be aquired through practice alone. Once the microscope is brought in, it should become your eyes and you should try to refrain from taking peeks into the operative field from the side. Rely on nursing staff to hand you instruments and place haemostasis aids, such as patties, within your field of vision so that they can be reached without taking your eye off the bleeding point. Be warned that minor haemorrhage, being magnified by the microscope, will appear torrential. However, the microscope will also help identify small bleeding points so that they can be controlled. If a bleeding point is difficult to find, a good tip is to follow the bleeding upstream (remember: blood runs down-hill) until it is identified. Figure 38 shows a typical view down an operative microscope.

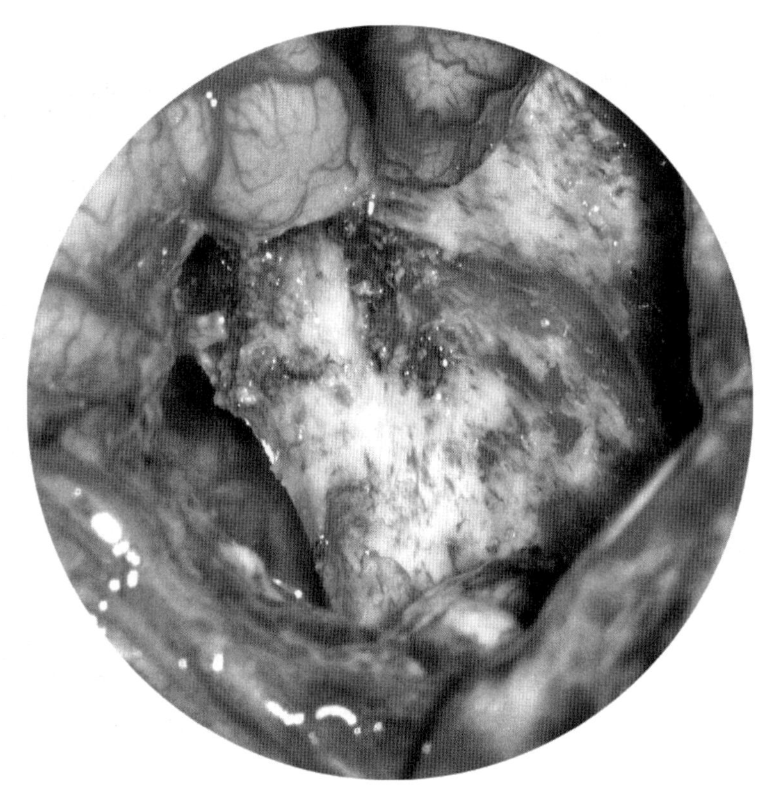

Figure 38. A typical view of an operative field as seen down an operating neurosurgical microscope.

The microscope is usually used with the surgeon in the seated position for cranial surgery and in the standing position for spinal surgery. A good chair with armrests is absolutely essential, as without armrests your arms will be unsupported. In cranial microsurgery only the forearms are usually supported.

Mastery of your tools is one of the cornerstones of good surgery. Familiarize yourself with the microscopes in your unit and try to practice using the controls and setting up the microscope when there is no operating going on.

NEW ADVANCES: IMAGE GUIDANCE SYSTEMS

Integration of the operating microscope into a frameless stereotactical navigational system is one of the most exciting advances in neurosurgery. Information on the angle of the micrsocope and the focal length

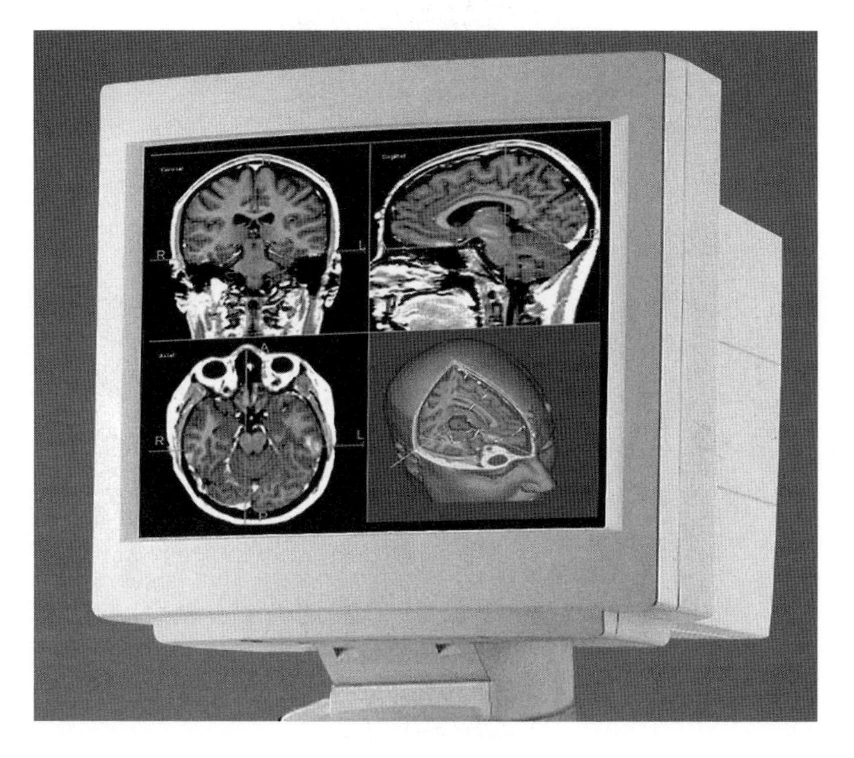

Figure 39. The type of reconstructed images as seen on a Carl Zeiss stereotactic navigational system.

can be digitalized and integrated with an infrared localising system. This information is compared with data from MR or CT scan imaging data that have been incorporated into the guidance system. The result is a displayed, reconstructed image that shows the surgeon where pathological tissue is located in relation both to normal tissues and to other operative equipment (see Figure 39).

12

Controversies and Evidence in Neurosurgery

CONTENTS

INTRODUCTION

The aim of this chapter is not to review systematically the evidence base in neurosurgery, nor is it to identify every area of controversy in neurosurgery. We have selected a few topics that often crop up in discussions in morning meetings, in theatre, and on the wards. It is hoped that this chapter will give SHOs a basis on which to participate actively in these discussions.

PROPHYLACTIC ANTIBIOTICS IN NEUROSURGERY

The use of antibiotics in neurosurgery is widespread yet remains controversial due to the paucity of a solid evidence base. This reflects the difficulties in gathering data in this area of neurosurgery. For example, although in skull fractures with associated CSF leak the incidence of infection may be as high as 25%, the actual incidence of CSF leak is very low. This means that it is extremely difficult to undertake a proper prospective study to compare prophylactic antibiotic regimens with acute treatment of frank infection. The rationale for recommendations regarding the use of prophylactic antibiotics in neurosurgery tends to be based on assessments of the risk of infection, the likely organisms involved, and the penetration of the antibiotic to the site of infection (e.g., CSF penetration across the blood–brain barrier, or penetration of tissues in the surgical field).

The British Association of Antimicrobial Chemotherapists has established working parties to review the evidence on the use of antibiotics in all surgical specialties and its web-pages provide a useful resource of summaries and conclusions regarding antibiotic prophylaxis (www.bsac.org.uk/pyxis/). The working party on neurosurgical infections looked at skull fractures, CSF leaks, and neurosurgical procedures (clean, non-implant procedure; clean–contaminated surgical procedures, e.g., breach of a cranial sinus or naso-/oro-pharynx; CSF and shunt surgery).

SKULL FRACTURES AND CSF LEAK

Up to 25% of patients with CSF leaks associated with base-of-skull fractures will develop infections. The most common organism causing post-traumatic meningitis is *Pneumococcus spp*. There are certain situations, however, when *S. aureus* and Gram –ve bacilli will be causative organisms, namely: depressed skull fractures; penetrating brain injuries; patients who have already been on antibiotics for other reasons; and those who have been in hospital for a length of time. The use of prophylactic antibiotics in skull fractures with CSF leak is not supported, due to the paucity of conclusive evidence. However, the situation with penetrating brain injury is somewhat different, as there appears to be a particularly high risk of infection, including meningitis, osteomyelitis and cerebral abscess formation. Although evidence is not available, because appropriate randomized controlled trials have not yet been performed, prophylactic antibiotic use has become widespread routine practice. This seems to be supported by lower rates of infection recorded in studies conducted after World War II, compared with the results of earlier studies (Arabi et al., 2001). Due to the wide spectrum of organisms that appear to be responsible for infection in penetrating brain injury, broad-spectrum antibiotics tend to be recommended, such as 5 days of co-amoxiclav 1.2 g IV tds, or 5 days cefuroxime 1.5 g IV stat followed by 750 mg IV tds plus metronidazole 500 mg IV tds.

NEUROSURGICAL PROCEDURES

Clean, non-implant surgery

The British Association of Antimicrobial Chemotherapists Working Party concluded that there is a significant amount of evidence to show that antibiotic prophylaxis may be beneficial for clean non-implant surgery.

Antibiotics were recommended on the basis of appropriate spectrum of activity (efficacy against likely pathogens: *S. aureus*; other Gram +ve cocci; and Gram –ve bacilli), as well as penetration to the surgical field. An example regimen would be cefuroxime 1.5 g IV at induction of anaesthesia followed by further 750 mg doses every 3 h during operation. It was concluded that there was no evidence to support prolonging prophylaxis beyond the time of surgery. However, there is no real evidence the other way either, and a commonly used regimen includes two further doses of cefuroxime at 8-h intervals following the first dose at induction.

Clean–contaminated surgery

The British Association of Antimicrobial Chemotherapists Working Party concluded that the case for antibiotic prophylaxis was supported by available evidence, and recommendations included the use of cefuroxime and metronidazole at induction and for the duration of surgery, but no longer.

CSF shunt surgery

The British Association of Antimicrobial Chemotherapists Working Party could not find any evidence that antibiotic prophylaxis is beneficial in shunt surgery. Due to the potentially devastating consequences of shunt infection, however, the large majority of neurosurgeons will elect to use antibiotics. The working party, therefore, proposed the following guidance on antibiotic choice, based on organisms commonly responsible for shunt infection. Shunt infections are most commonly due to coagulase-negative *Staphylococcus spp.* (90%), *S. aureus* (>20%), and aerobic Gram –ve bacilli (>10%). Theoretically at least, vancomycin and gentamicin would be effective, but neither enters the CSF well from the peripheral circulation, and they would, therefore, have to be given intraventricularly. It is, however, common for neurosurgeons to soak and prime shunts with gentamicin solution before insertion. Many people also use a cefuroxime regimen to cover external infection from the wound.

Arabi, B, Alden, T, Chesnut R et al.. Antibiotic prophylaxis for penetrating brain injury. J Trauma 2001; 51: S34–S40. This is an excellent review of the evidence supporting the recommendation to use antibiotic prophylaxis in penetrating brain injury. This article can be viewed on-line at www.neurosurgery.org/trauma/guidelines/.

www.bsac.org.uk/pyxis/ Website summarising findings of a Working Party of the British Association of Antimicrobial Chemotherapists into Neurosurgical Infection.

ANTICONVULSANT THERAPY IN SEVERE TRAUMATIC BRAIN INJURY

The use of anticonvulsants, and phenytoin in particular, is widespread practice in patients who suffer seizures following traumatic brain injury. More controversial, however, is the use of phenytoin prophylactically to prevent seizures occurring, especially when one has to balance the potentially harmful adverse effects of medication.

Up to 50% of patients suffering a penetrating brain injury will develop seizures. Of these, approximately 10% will show seizures in the first week following injury and by 2 years 80% of those who are going to fit will have done so (Pruitt, 2001). A seizure occurring in the first week is referred to as an early post-traumatic seizure (EPTS); seizures occurring after this period are referred to as delayed post-traumatic seizure (DPTS). Studies looking at antiepileptic use in brain injury usually consider the effectiveness of anticonvulsants on EPTS and DPTS separately. When considering the use of anticonvulsants to prevent DPTS it is important to realise that 95% of patients suffering penetrating brain injury will remain seizure free if they have not suffered a seizure in the first 3 years (Weiss et al., 1986).

The published evidence is limited and conflicting. Where trials have been conducted there is considerable disagreement regarding the validity of the methodology. For a good recent example of two conflicting opinions, read the correspondence between Professors Chang and Lowenstein of Harvard Medical School and Professor Latronico of the University of Brescia, Italy (Chang and Lowenstein, 2003). Basically, there is one body of opinion suggesting that phenytoin is effective in reducing EPTS but not DPTS, and another body of opinion that holds that phenytoin is lacking in efficacy in both situations. There are even two conflicting trials that back up each point of view. Temkin et al. (1990) undertook a randomized, double-blind study of 404 patients at risk of post-traumatic seizures; 208 received phenytoin within 24 h of injury and 196 received placebo. A 3.6% incidence EPTS was reported in the phenytoin group, compared to 14.2% in the placebo group. No effect on DPTS was found. The authors concluded that phenytoin is beneficial only in the first week after severe head injury. This is in contradiction to the finding of an earlier, similar trial undertaken by Young et al. (1973) which involved 244 patients, but in which no benefit was found for phenytoin in either EPTS or DPTS.

It would appear from the evidence so far that, if there is any benefit from phenytoin, it will be only in EPTS, and so administration for a longer period of time would not be necessary. However, the existing evidence is there to help in the decision-making process, and it is appropriate, when considering anticonvulsants in individual cases, to take account of the extent to which their situation resembles those of patients included in the existing trials. Individual Consultants working side-by-side within the same neurosurgical unit may differ in their practice with regard to prophylactic phenytoin. It is an interesting exercise to enquire as to their reasons, as they will have a wealth of clinical experience which will have shaped their practice. So far, there is little evidence concerning the degree to which the nature of penetrating brain injury influences the risk of post-traumatic seizure, e.g., the site of cortical injury, the presence of a foreign body, or infection. This does not mean to say that such factors are not relevant, but only that there just has not been a study big enough to find any answers.

Chang BS, Lowenstein DG. Practice parameter: antiepileptic drug prophylaxis in severe traumatic brain injury. Neurology 2003; 60: 10–16 (See associated correspondence).
Pruit B. Antiseizure prophylaxis for penetrating brain injury. J Trauma 2001; 51: S41–S44.
Temkin NR, Dikmen SS, Wilensky AJ, Keihm J, Chabal S, Winn HR. A randomised, double-blinded study of phenytoin for the prevention of post-traumatic seizures. N Engl J Med 1990; 8: 497–502.
Weiss GH, Salazar AM, Vance SC, Grafman JH, Jabbain B. Predicting posttraumatic epilepsy in penetrating head injury. Arch Neurol 1986; 43: 771–773.
Young B, Rapp RP, Norton JA, Haack D, Tibbs PA, Bean JR. Failure of prophylactically administered phenytoin to prevent early posttraumatic seizures. J Neurosurg 1983; 58: 231–235.

STEROIDS IN HEAD INJURY

The use of steroids in head injury has become more topical recently with the advent of the CRASH trial that is currently under way. Studies to date have been relatively small. A comprehensive review of the randomized trials was undertaken by Alderson and Roberts (1997). They found that, even when all patient data from the trials was combined, the numbers of patients involved was only a little over 2000 and there seemed to be only a 2% reduction in mortality with the use of steroids, and this was not statistically significant. Nevertheless, a 2% reduction in mortality would represent a large number of lives saved due to the millions of deaths from severe head injury each year. This has been the incentive of the CRASH trial which aims to include >10 000 and hopefully >20 000 patients. This should be a sufficient sample size to establish whether or not steroids are of any benefit in severe head injury. The details of the trial are published on the web (www.crash.lshtm.ac.uk).

The majority of patients in the CRASH trial will be treated outwith the neurosurgical unit. However, the trial will undoubtedly be discussed when head injury patients are transferred in who have been included in the trial. Opinions will differ greatly regarding steroid use. It is particularly pertinent to consider the implications of a reduction in mortality in severe head injury. One step up in outcome from death is severe morbidity. Is death really always the worst outcome? If the use of steroids in severe head injury is to be accepted by many neurosurgeons, then studies will have to show a reduction in severe morbidity.

Alderson P and Roberts I. Corticosteroids in acute traumatic brain injury: systematic review of randomised controlled trials. Br Med J 1997; 314: 1855–1859.
www.crash.lshtm.ac.uk

STEROIDS IN SPINAL CORD INJURY

Several clinical trials have been done to evaluate the use of steroids in spinal cord injury. However, this treatment modality remains controversial and practice differs between clinicians and centres.

A Cochrane review of the evidence (Bracken, 2000) found that too few studies had been conducted in this area, but that a meta-analysis of three trials (one in North America, one in Japan, and one in France) showed some apparent benefit for methyl prednisolone. However, there has been much discussion in the literature regarding the methodology of these trials. Improved outcome in motor function was seen at 1 year, provided that methyl prednisolone was given within 8 h of injury and in the following regimen: (1) 30 mg/kg bolus; (2) an infusion of 5.4 mg/kg/h for a further 23 h. It was also possible that further motor improvement might occur if infusion was continued for a total of 48 h. A more recent review found that, although neurological improvement was seen with methyl prednisolone, there was no effect on overall mortality (Spencer and Bazarian, 2003). All reviewers indicate that further studies are required to establish the efficacy of corticosteroids in spinal cord injury, and appropriate treatment regimens for their use.

Bracken MB. Steroids for acute spinal injury. Cochrane Database Syst Rev 2000; 2: CD001046.
Spencer MT, Bazarian JJ. Are corticosteroids effective in traumatic spinal cord injury? Ann Emerg Med 2003; 41: 410–413.

ISSUES IN SUBARACHNOID HAEMORRHAGE

NIMODIPINE TO PREVENT SECONDARY CEREBRAL ISCHAEMIA

Secondary ischaemia is a significant cause of poor outcome in SAH, and may be due to vasospasm. A double-blind, placebo-controlled trial involving 554 patients (Pickard et al., 1980) found that the calcium antagonist, nimodipine, seemed to be effective in reducing cerebral infarction and the incidence of poor outcome at 3 months in SAH patients. A recent Cochrane review (Rinkel et al., 2002) looked at the evidence gathered subsequently from 11 trials and concluded that the evidence was in favour of the use of nimodipine. However, the evidence is only for oral nimodipine given 4-hourly, and not for IV regimens. In addition, the Cochrane review indicated that the efficacy of calcium antagonists might not be as clear-cut for patients with established ischaemia or with a poor initial grade of SAH. Further studies may reveal improved dosing regimens and consider the efficacy of calcium antagonists other than nimodipine.

Pickard JD, Murray GD, Illingworth R et al. Br Med J 1989; 298: 636–640.
Rinkel GJ, Feigh VL, Alagra A, Vermeulen M, Van Gijn J. Calcium antagonists for anuerysal subarachnoid haemorrhage. Cochrane Database Syst Rev 2002; 4: CD000277.

ENDOVASCULAR COILING *VERSUS* SURGERY

Good clinical trials are rumoured to be rare in surgery. However, you should be aware of one particularly good neurosurgical trial that was reported recently. This is the ISAT trial (International Subarachnoid Aneurysm Trial, 2002) which compared the safety and efficacy of endovascular coiling of aneurysms with that of surgical clipping. This randomized, mulicentre trial was undertaken in Europe, and 2143 patients were enrolled. The ISAT group reported that coiling appeared to be safe and that its efficacy was significantly better than surgical clipping, in terms of survival free of disability at 1 year. Follow-up of patients in the trial is still underway. The trial has not been without its critics, however. Some observers have argued that, although the ISAT group showed that coiling was safe compared to clipping, the evidence was not as convincing for efficacy (Leung et al., 2003). Others have argued that there is an expertise bias in favour of endovascular interventionalists (Britz et al., 2003). The response of the ISAT group to such criticisms can be read in the literature (Molyneaux and Kerr, 2003). Further follow-up of data in the ISAT trial are due to be published in the near future and will be well worth looking out for.

Britz GW, Newell DW, West A, Lam A. The ISAT trial. Lancet 2003; 361: 431–432.
International Subarachnoid Haemorrhage Collaborative Group. International Subarachnoid Aneurysm Trial (ISAT) of neurosurgical clipping versus endovascular coiling in 2143 patients with ruptured intracranial aneurysms: a randomised trial. Lancet 2002; 360: 1267–1274.
Leung CHS, Poon WS, Yu LM. The ISAT trial. Lancet 2003; 361: 430–431.
Molyneux A, Kerr A. The ISAT trial. Lancet 2003; 361: 432.

PERIOPERATIVE ANTICONVULSANT PROPHYLAXIS

Although the administration of prophylactic anticonvulsant medication has been accepted practice for aneurysmal surgery for many years, the benefits of these medications need to be balanced against the risk of adverse reactions with these drugs. A retrospective study (Baker et al., 1995) found that the incidence of seizures following craniotomy for aneurysm repair was low, and it was concluded that the administration of prophylactic phenytoin was necessary only for the first 7 days postoperatively. There seems to be a paucity of strong evidence for the prolonged use of prophylactic anticonvulsants in SAH.

Baker CJ, Prestigiacamo CJ, Solomon RA. Short-term perioperative anticonvulsant prophylaxis for the surgical treatment of low-risk patients with intracranial aneurysms. Neurosurgery 1995; 37: 863–871.

TIMING OF SURGERY FOR SUBARACHNOID HAEMORRHAGE

The timing of subarachnoid surgery is one of the most contentious issues in neurosurgery. In some cases, the presence of a large, life-threatening clot, demands early craniotomy. Indeed, it can be argued that, on theoretical grounds, there are good reasons to operate in the first 2–3 days following rupture, e.g., the risk of re-bleeding will be reduced and protection of the aneurysm allows for more aggressive treatment of vasospasm. However, there are equally good arguments against early surgery, e.g., the amount of blood and brain oedema present immediately after a bleed makes surgery more difficult (due to difficulty retracting the parenchyma) and operative mortality is higher. Although there have been a number of studies looking at this issue, there is still no consensus (Milhorat and Krautheim 1986; Kassel et al., 1990; de Gans et al., 2002).

de Gans K, Nieuwkamp DJ, Rinkel GJ, Algra A. Timing of aneurysm surgery in subarachnoid hemorrhage: a systematic review of the literature. Neurosurgery 2002; 50: 336–340.
Kassell NF, Torner JC, Jane JA. The international cooperative study on the timing of aneurysm surgery. Part 2: surgical results. J Neurosurg 1990; 73: 37–47.
Milhorat TH, Krautheim M. Results of early and delayed operations for ruptured intracranial aneurysms in two series of 100 consequetive patients. Surg Neurol 1986; 26:123–128.

THIOPENTONE TO CONTROL ICP IN SEVERE HEAD INJURY

The use of barbiturates, such as thiopentone, to control ICP remains controversial, particularly because their administration prolongs the ICU stay of severely brain damaged patients, without necessarily improving their clinical outcome. It was shown that the administration of barbiturates is effective in lowering ICP (Shapiro et al., 1979). Although it is widely accepted that control of ICP improves survival and outcome in severe head injury, there is conflicting evidence that the use of high-dose barbiturates achieves this aim (Rea and Lockswold, 1983; Ward et al., 1985).

Rea GL, Rockswold GL. Barbiturate therapy in uncontrolled hypertension. Neurosurgery 1983; 12: 401–404.
Shapiro HM, Wyte SR, Loeser J. Barbiturate augmented hypothermia for reduction of persistent intracranial hypertension. J Neurosurg 1979; 40: 90–100.
Ward JD, Becker DP, Miller JD et al. Failure of prophylactic barbiturate coma in the treatment of severe head injury. J Neurosurg 1985; 62: 383–388.

13
Commonly Used Scoring Systems in Neurosurgery

CONTENTS

THE GLASGOW COMA SCALE

Table 2 is a modified version of the Glasgow Coma Scale.

Table 2. The Modified Glasgow Coma Scale.

Score	Eye opening (max = 4)	Verbal response (max = 5	Motor response (max = 6))
6	–	–	Obeys
5	–	Orientated	Localizes
4	Spontaneous	Confused	Withdraws
3	To speech	Inappropriate	Flexion (decorticate)
2	To pain	Incomprehensible	Extension (decerebrate)
1	None	None	None

Teasdale G, Jennett B. Assessment of coma and impaired consciousness: a practical scale. Lancet 1974; ii: 81-84.

THE GLASGOW OUTCOME SCALE

Table 3 is a modified summary of the Glasgow Outcome Scale (GOS), which was designed for the assessment of outcome in head injuries. The GOS is a valuable and established research tool. When critically evaluating new treatment modalities for head injury that are reported to produce improvements in the GOS, it is necessary to consider exactly what that means for the patient. For example, a treatment modality might be shown to improve the GOS in 90% of patients; however, if the improvement equates to improvements from a GOS of 1 to 2, i.e., from death to a persistent vegetative state, then it is worth considering the implications for the patient. Is death always the worst outcome?

Table 3. The Glasgow Outcome Scale (modified).

Score	Description of patient
5	Normal life
4	Mild disability, able to perform basic activities of daily life independently, but not able to resume previously normal life
3	Severely disabled and dependent
2	Persistent vegetative state
1	Death

Jennett B, Bond M. The assessment of outcome after severe brain damage: a practical scale. Lancet 1975; i: 480-484.

WFNS GRADE OF SUBARACHNOID HAEMORRHAGE

Table 4. The WFNS grading scale for subarachnoid haemorrhage.

WFNS grade	GSC	Focal deficit (aphasia, hemiparesis)
0 (unruptured aneurysm)	–	–
1	15	None
2	13-14	None
3	13-14	Present
4	7-12	None or present
5	3-6	None or present

Drake C G. Report of World Federation of Neurological Surgeons Committee on a universal subarachnoid haemorrhage grading scale. J Neurosurg 1988; 68: 985-986.

FISHER GRADE OF CT FINDINGS IN SUBARACHNOID HAEMORRHAGE

A poor Fisher grade correlates with increased risk of vasospasm.

Table 5. The Fisher scale for grading CT findings in subarachnoid haemorrhage.

Fisher grade	Blood on CT
1	None detected
2	Diffuse or vertical layers[a] <1 mm thick
3	Localized clot or vertical layer >1 mm thick
4	Intracerebral or intraventricular clot

[a] Vertical layers refers to subarachnoid spaces, e.g., intrahemisphere fissure.

Fisher C M, Kistler J P, Davis J M. Relation of cerebral vasospasm to subarachnoid haemorrhage visualized by CT scanning. Neurosurgery 1980; 6: 1-9.

MRC SCORE FOR MUSCLE STRENGTH ASSESSMENT

Table 6. The MRC scale for grading muscle strength.

Grade	Strength
0	No contraction
1	Flicker
2	Moves if gravity eliminated
3	Gravity overcome
4	Moves against resistance
5	Normal strength

KARNOFSKY SCORE

The Karnofsky score was devised as a clinical and research tool to grade the functional status in cancer patients. The maximum and best score is 100, which implies normal functioning. Lower scores imply varying degrees of symptomatology, disability and sickness. The lowest score is 0 and implies death.

Table 7. The Karnofsky performance score.

Condition and percentage	Comments
A. *Able to carry on normal activity and to work. No special care needed*	
100	Normal, no complaints, no evidence of disease.
90	Able to carry on normal activity, minor signs or symptoms of disease.
80	Normal activity with effort, some signs or symptoms of disease.
B. *Unable to work. Able to live at home, care for most personal needs A varying degree of assistance is needed.*	
70	Cares for self. Unable to carry on normal activity or to do active work.
60	Requires occasional assistance, but is able to care for most of own needs.
50	Disease may be progressing rapidly. Requires considerable assistance and frequent medical care.
C. *Unable to care for self. Requires equivalent of institutional or hospital care.*	
40	Disabled. Requires special care and assistance.
30	Severely disabled, hospitalization is indicated although death is not imminent.
20	Hospitalization necessary, very sick, active supportive treatment necessary.
10	Moribund, fatal processses progressing rapidly.
0	Dead.

Karnofsky DA, Burchenal JH. The clinical evaluation of chemotherapeutic agents in cancer. In: Macleod CM, ed. Evaluation of chemotherapy agents. New York: Columbia University Press, 1949: 191-205.
www.acsu.buffalo.edu/~drstall/assessmenttools.html

FURTHER READING

Crockard A, Haywards R, Hoff JT, eds. *Neurosurgery: the Scientific Basis of Clinical Practice*, 3rd edn. Oxford: Blackwell Science, 2001.

Greenberg MS. *Handbook of Neurosurgery*, 5th edn. Berlin: Thieme, 2001.

Jennett B, Lindsay KW. *An Introduction to Neurosurgery*, 5th edn. London: Butterworth Heinemann, 1994.

Kaye AH. *Essential Neurosurgery*, 2nd edn. Edinburgh: Churchill Livingstone, 1997.

Lindsay KW, Bone I. *Neurology and Neurosurgery Illustrated*, 3rd edn. Edinburgh: Churchill Livingstone, 1997.

Moore AJ, Newell D, eds. *Neurosurgery*. Berlin: Springer Verlag, 2003.

Patten J. *Neurological Differential Diagnosis*, 2nd edn. Berlin: Springer Verlag, 2001.

Tindall GT, Cooper PR, Barrow DL, eds. *Practice of Neurosurgery*. London: Lippincott, Williams & Wilkins, 1996

Winn RH, ed. *Youman's Neurological Surgery*, 5th edn. New York: W. B. Saunders, 2003.

ABBREVIATIONS

A&E	Accident and emergency
ACA	Anterior cerebral artery
Acomm	Anterior communicating artery
ACTH	Adreocorticotrophic hormone
ADH	Antidiuretic hormone
AF	Atrial fibrillation
AP	Anteroposterior
ASDH	Acute subdural haemorrhage/haematoma
ATLS	Advanced trauma life support
AVM	Arteriovenous malformation
BA	Basilar artery
cACA(A2)	Contralateral anterior cerebral artery A2 segment
CCrISP	Care of the critically ill surgical patient
CNS	Central nervous system
Coag screen	Coagulation screening 81
CPP	Cerebral perfusion pressure
CRASH	Corticosteroid Randomisation After Significant Head Injury
CRP	C-reactive protein
CSDH	Chronic subdural haematoma
CSF	Cerebrospinal fluid
CSW	Cerebral salt wasting
CT	Computerized tomography
CTA	CT angiography
CVA	Cerebrovascular accident
CVP	Central venous pressure
CXR	Chest X-ray
DDAVP	1-d-amino-8-D-arginine vasopressin
DI	Diabetes insipidus
DIND	Delayed ischaemic neurological deficit
DPTS	Delayed post-traumatic seizure
DVT	Deep-vein thrombosis
EAM	External auditory meatus
EDH	Epidural haemorrhage/haematoma
EEG	Electroencephalogram
EMG	Electromyography
EPTS	Early post-traumatic seizure
ESR	Erythrocyte sedimentation rate
ET	Endotracheal
EVD	External ventricular drain
Ex	Examination
FBC	Full blood count
FSH	Follicle-stimulating hormone

GBM	Glioblastoma multiforme
GCS	Glasgow Coma Scale
GH	Growth hormone
β-HCG	Human chorionic gonadotrophin
HDU	High-dependency unit
Hx	History
iACA(A2)	Ispilateral anterior cerebral artery A2 segment
ICA	Internal carotid artery
ICP	Intracranial pressure
ICU	Intensive care unit
IgF1	Immunoglobulin F1
INR	International normalized ratio
ISAT	International Subarachnoid Aneurysm Trial
IQ	Intelligence quotient
IV	Intravenous
LAICA	Left anterior inferior cerebellar artery
LAT	Locum Appointment for Training
LFT	Liver function tests
LH	Luteinizing hormone
LICA	Left internal carotid artery
LP	Lumbar puncture
LPICA	Left posterior inferior cerebellar artery
LVA	Left vertebral artery
MAP	Mean arterial pressure
MCA	Middle cerebral artery
MI	Myocardial infarction
MR	Magnetic resonance
MRA	Magnetic resonance angiography
MRC	Medical Research Council
MRI	Magnetic resonance imaging
NF1	Neurofibromatosis type 1
NF2	Neurofibromatosis type 2
obs	Observations
ophth.a	Ophthalmic artery
Pcomm	Posterior communicating artery
PE	Pulmonary embolism
PNET	Primitive neuro-ectodermal tumours
PR	Per rectum
PSA	Prostate-specific antigen
RICA	Right internal carotid artery
RPCA	Right posterior cerebellar artery
RSCA	Right superior cerebellar artery
RTA	Road traffic accident
RVA	Right vertebral artery

SAH	Subarachnoid haemorrhage
sats	Haemaglobin oxygen saturation
SCIWORA	Spinal cord injury without radiological abnormality
SDH	Subdural haemorrhage
SHO	Senior House Officer
SIADH	Syndrome of inappropriate antidiuretic hormone secretion
SM	Spetzler-Martin
SpR	Specialist Registrar
TEDs	Thromboembolic-deterrant stockings
U & E	Urea and electrolytes
WCC	White cell count
WFNS	World Federation of Neurosurgeons